Strong Medicine

Health Politics for the Twenty-First Century

Steve Iliffe

LAWRENCE AND WISHART
LONDON

Lawrence and Wishart Limited
39 Museum Street
London WC1A 1LQ

First published 1988
© Steve Iliffe, 1988

Photoset in North Wales by
Derek Doyle & Associates, Mold, Clwyd.
Printed and bound in Great Britain by
Billing & Sons, Worcester

STRONG MEDICINE

For Ursula and Paul

Contents

Acknowledgements

This book is based on three articles, one of which appeared in *Critical Social Policy*, No. 14, Winter 1985-86, and two which appeared in *Marxism Today* in October 1986 and Febuary 1988. I am grateful to Chris Phillipson for his prompting, to Martin Jacques for his merciless but essential editorial approach, and to Stephen Hayward for firm encouragement.

Introduction

Above all, it is the left, not the right,
which should be working, in the name of
social progress, for the abandonment of the
principle of universal entitlement to
public provision regardless of need.

David Selbourne, *New Statesman*, 16 October 1987

If the leaders of the Labour Party have a plan to save the National Health Service, they are keeping it to themselves. Yet the situation warrants that overworked word 'crisis', for the continued survival of the health service in its present form now seems unlikely. Thatcherism may be close to breaking the central institution of the welfare state, and Labour's most popular nationalised industry.

The health of the nation has improved enormously for some since 1948, but not for everyone. The experience of health and illness of the unskilled working class has hardly changed since the NHS was founded, but the more affluent and powerful have added life to years and years to life. The differences in experience between the extremes of wealth and poverty are so great that no one system of medical care seems able to satisfy such different needs and such diverging expectations. We are moving towards parallel health services for different populations, perhaps a three- or four-tier service to match a nation divided into the affluent and secure, the better-off but insecure, and the poor. As this book argues, this is occurring because of material changes in health experience and the lack of a political alternative to Conservatism, and not through simple Tory ill will and the manipulation of an undemocratic government machine.

What are the possible futures? What can the left expect to achieve whilst the Conservatives remain in office, and what could a Labour goverment do with, or for, the National Health Service? If only we knew! Without a real grasp of what is happening now, and with a background of crying disaster at every change that threatened the existing service, the left has lost its way. Increasingly, socialists are forced to defend an institution that was designed for a society that no longer exists, and which until very recently we criticised incessantly for its shortcomings. (There are honourable exceptions to this rule, but they prove it true, and will have to wait for the history of this period to be written before their lack of influence on political parties and trade unions can be measured exactly.)

This book tries to explain the left's failure to understand and control the health service it created, and looks at the possibilities for renewing the NHS and creating a new kind of welfare state. It does so in ways that may be unsettling; readers accustomed to the bumpy ride of current politics will take them in their stride.

The first part, 'The End of the Beginning?', assesses the current political crisis of the NHS and speculates on possible medium- and long-term outcomes by using three 'future histories' in which similar events combine in different ways to produce very different results.

Part 2, 'The Erosion of Principles', describes the origins and subsequent modification of the main features of the NHS – a comprehensive service free at the time of need, financed from general taxation – and asks a number of questions. What did these features within the political culture of post-war Britain, how were they interpreted by the left and the labour movement in subsequent decades, and how do they fit into the politics of Labour today?

The third part outlines the twin crises within the NHS. The first crisis stems from the recession within the international economy, and the attempts of Conservative governments to escape from it. The second crisis is within medical practice itself, appearing as an escalation of costs without a comparable increase in cure, care or prevention.

'Orthodoxies and Heresies', Part 4, discusses the likely

impact of continued technological development on medicine and health care, in the context of a new model of care, the 'life cycle' welfare state.

Notes at the end of each part develop points, give sources and contain further details. There are three appendices: an outline of the contents of a computer programme for a personal medical record held on a floppy disc; a 'Patient's Charter' listing possible future statutory responsibilities of Health Authorities towards citizens; and targets for NHS activity, derived from the World Health Organisation's programme, 'Health for All by the Year 2000'.

The conclusion is optimistic, and contradicts David Selbourne. A new kind of welfare state is waiting to be created, on the basis of universal provision. Rebuilding the National Health Service on modern foundations may take us towards that new concept of welfare and into a new society.

Steve Iliffe,
24 March 1987

1   The End of the Beginning?

The bone marrow unit at Westminster Children's Hospital deals not with leukaemia but with 50 other previously fatal genetic diseases. A bone marrow transplant costs £16,000 and half of that cost is met by charity ... [the] unit has seven beds which require 36 paediatric nurses. The unit has only six nurses because of the poor wages ... As a result only two beds can be used. Instead of 40 bone marrow transplants a year, 15 are being carried out. The waiting list holds the names of 50 children.

It's been a bad fortnight for the National Health Service but a good one for charity balls. Six in London in ten days. Cancer, physical disabilities, leukaemia ... One night can reap £30,000 and more ...

'If it's kids, I'll spend,' says a jovial man popping *petits fours* into his mouth like peanuts. He reckons he's 'shelled out' around £250 this evening.

... the contribution of many charity ball givers is proportionally a smaller slice in terms of their income than, say, that given by an old age pensioner.

Yvonne Roberts, 'If You've Got it, Flaunt it', *New Statesman*, 18 December 1987

All politicians love babies, especially before elections. That is why Margaret Thatcher is so unusual. Her interest in a baby boy waiting for cardiac surgery in a West Midlands hospital in the autumn of 1987 came *after* the Conservatives' triumph in the June General Election. She had no obvious need for the boy, so why did he catch her eye? It may have been real concern, but that seems unlikely given the plight of so many, young and old, who have experienced the impact of Conservatism's 'hard decisions' on the NHS. Concern seems an even less probable explanation for the actions of a Prime Minister whose government has used mass unemployment as an economic lever and as a political weapon.

One million more children were living on Supplementary Benefit in 1987 than in 1978, yet it was a Conservative government that rejected the Black Report's 1980 plan to abolish child poverty.[1] The growth in poverty affecting children is likely to widen the class gap in the take-up of preventive services, in concepts of self-care, in seeking professional advice early in the course of illness and in exposure to hazardous experiences. Although the class differences in child health have been less marked than those amongst adults, the early damage to health experienced by children from poor families will, on past experience, establish patterns of ill health that persist into adult life.[2] Changes in health care policy encouraged by Thatcher's administrations may be making things worse for the poor. For example, the shift towards community care and 'prevention' has meant an intensification of the home workload of parents – primarily women – whilst professionals take on roles of assessment and surveillance.[3]

Perhaps the close attention of media lenses sharpened her vision and shook her confidence. After all, before the 1983 General Election the Prime Minister herself had proclaimed that the NHS was safe in Conservative hands. After that victory she had added that she had no more intention of dismantling the health service than she had of dismantling the nation's defences. Now an ill child and his worried parents threatened those boasts. No one could accuse the boy of shroud-waving, and neither he nor his parents were politically motivated agitators upsetting the decent professionals keen to get on with their work.

Against a background clamour for more resources for the health service, and an apparently unending stream of informed criticism of the government's stewardship of the NHS, the personal story of one baby made abstract politics tangible and powerful. The boy's desperate family voiced the anger and fear of hundreds of parents whose children were in the same plight, and hundreds of thousands of others who could blame their long wait for treatment or poor care in overworked hospitals on a mean and indifferent government.

At long last, the National Health Service and its users were turning on the Tories. Health Authorities were threatened with legal action by their professional employees, who had learned mutiny from porters and cleaners engaged in earlier disputes over privatisation, and by users like the parents of the baby boy needing cardiac surgery.[4] Television documentaries scanned overcrowded waiting rooms and interviewed health workers who were scathing about official assurance that all was well within the NHS. Stern surgeons, flanked as ever by supportive nurses, spread petition pages for the cameras, with Downing Street as the backdrop.

Exposing the Bones

Little of this was new. The NHS was underfunded in 1983, when Margaret Thatcher insisted that it was safe in Conservative hands. There had been petitions by the hundred, sad stories of treatment refused and old, frail people decanted from place to place, demonstrations and occupations, angry fights in Health Authority meetings, white coated protestors on television and press coverage by the column mile. So why in the autumn of 1987 was the NHS hot news, and why did so much protest reach our screens and papers? Was it not all there before, but unattended by the media?

Some was and some was not. Trimming the fat from the NHS budget has done more than make the service lean. It has bared the bones of NHS medicine, the 'acute' hospitals, and launched a wave of professional anger. Budget cuts that had whittled away the family planning clinics and community nursing services were bad, but not bad enough for the kind of political response we began to see late in 1987. Speedy discharge of hospital patients caused problems for them, and sometimes for the hospitals when they were readmitted more ill than before, yet it was all tolerable for those with higher priorities.[5] Closure of long-stay mental illness beds might produce local scandals, badly damaged men and women surviving in solitary, squalid accommodation or opting out of shabby, lonely bedsitters to live rough, but none of it interfered too much with the essence of our health service, the coronary care units and the operating theatres and the incubators for tiny babies. Of course, there were waiting lists and shortages and queues, but not everywhere, and not if you knew how to use the system, and everything held together somehow.[6]

Until the autumn of 1987. Then there were insufficient beds in coronary care, too few nurses to run theatres, more tiny babies than incubators and no trimmable luxury services like child psychiatry or psychosexual counselling big enough to close the huge gap in the budget. Whole wards had to go, then whole hospitals.[7]

At this point the powerful hospital specialists who had wept at every cut, but who had also counselled caution and withdrawal to the next barricade, glanced behind to find – nothing. For many hospital consultants, particularly those in London teaching hospitals, the barricade they were at looked like the last. Their slots in the new commercial hospitals were *pieds-à-terre*, not homes. There were no research departments, massive back-up facilities or large junior teams on call to match those of the NHS, even in the biggest commercial emporia. The NHS remained the base, the launching pad for almost all clinical practice and scientific medicine. It paid badly by comparison with the commercial sector, but in 1987 it had no rivals.

Professional Power

Self-interest is not the whole story behind the professionals' campaigns for the NHS in the autumn and winter, but it is a large part. That does not mean that the protests were not genuine. 'Patient care' had been harmed, people were suffering because of government policy, and those who cared for them were angry. Their work is important, the help they give is necessary, often vital, and those in their care are (in the main) grateful for a good service well performed. Yet we need to repeat the question – what was new? The answer is that some patients, some problems and some professionals are more important than others. Our eyes are drawn to the baby in the incubator more often than to the dement in the wheelchair, and we listen to the surgeon more attentively than we do to the geriatrician. The political crisis around the NHS has revealed political priorities that have governed the health service for decades, and which are shared across different strata of society, across different age groups and across the political spectrum.

For a time this did not matter: there was a crisis and it had to be resolved. In the winter of 1987-88 it was not clear who would do this, and how. When a thousand senior figures in the medical profession signed a petition supporting the demand of the pressure group 'Hospital Alert' for extra NHS funding, was the government's intransigence dented at all? How much impact had opinion polls that showed the growth in public concern about the NHS? Did angry dispatch-box exchanges between Kinnock and Thatcher over health service cuts undermine Conservative confidence and credibility, or show Labour's powerlessness? Would the trade union movement intervene and, if so, how? What would the two studies of health service financing, undertaken by the King's Fund Institute and the Institute of Health Service Management, due out in the spring of 1988, conclude? Would the imminent official report on 'Community Care' be very critical of government policy, mildly critical, or simply even-handed? Would the Warnock review of embryo research policy be controversial, with serious implications for both the NHS and commercial medicine, or would it pass largely unnoticed? Would David Alton's Bill to reduce the abortion time-limit prompt an anti-abortion backlash, or would it be weakened in Parliamentary Committee and in the House of Lords. Even if it were passed, could it be contained by professional resistance, spur improvements in family planning services and gynaecology generally and so damage fewer women's lives than anticipated?

What Kind of Health Service?

Asking these questions measures the depths of the political crisis in health care, for the left had few answers during that winter of campaigning, and gained few in the following spring. The crisis of the health service was then and remains now a political crisis for the left as well as for the right. Those few socialists with apparent power to influence the course of events in the health service through the parliamentary opposition, in the trade unions, even within the DHSS and its Health Authorities continue to lack the guidance of a workable strategy.

We face a dilemma. What kind of health service do we want, and what is possible? A major theme of this book is that the current cash crisis in the health service is only the surface of the problem, and those now campaigning for the core of NHS medicine, the 'acute' hospitals, are fighting for that part of the service which absorbs ever greater amounts of public money. Solving today's problem only to face it again tomorrow seems foolish, yet most of the left sees NHS underfunding as the fundamental, or even the only, issue. The underlying subject of value for money in medical care has been left to the right and centre to debate and formulate, with the inevitable result that these political trends dominate in a period of economic and political change, leaving socialists to argue for the status quo.

Our hospital services are capable of absorbing a growing proportion of the NHS budget, as they have done in London since 1981 after a brief period in which community health services expanded, and of making health services absorb a greater proportion of national wealth, as seems to have happened throughout the industrialised societies of Northern and Western Europe, North America and Japan since the 1960s. The specialists who have entered the political conflict with such vigour are concerned to increase the resources at their disposal, and in the medium term are likely to consider any system of funding that will offer this prospect. In 1987 the NHS had no rivals as the main source of finance, but that situation may change. Rapid development of the commercial sector is unlikely to happen in an across-the-board way, but speedy growth of some services is possible and has happened with in vitro fertilisation (IVF), 'natural' childbirth and even therapy for alcohol and drug dependency. The long-term growth trend within the commercial sector could carry it to the point at which it becomes a serious rival to the public service as a source of funding for a wider range of specialist provision.

The consequences of the growth of specialist medical care are an important political issue. Whilst there is no doubt that there have been improvements in the quality of life for many, and in the quantity of life for some, as a result of this growth, there is no way that modern medicine can claim the main credit for our improved health. That does not mean that we do not need hospitals or health services, but it certainly means that future governments must use public resources more carefully than has been done in the past, particularly in a damaged economy and society in desperate need of renewal and repair.

This situation is likely to worsen rather than ease because we are entering a new phase of technological change within medicine that will transform medical care, but at great expense. New methods of investigating the ways in which our bodies work, and of diagnosing and treating disease, particularly cancers, are now appearing. Their impact upon us will be great, although almost inevitably less than promised by their enthusiastic supporters. From past experience of technical innovation in medicine the research, development and application costs of new advances are likely to be greater than expected.

Strategy Wanted

Those socialists who think they have a strategy that will allow us to develop a national health service out of the current dilemma are impotent, separated from power sources by their outdated assumptions and expectations. This applies not only to the ultra-left, for whom impotence is a defining characteristic, but also to the mainstream. We do not lack practical ideas about particular approaches and kinds of service, but we do lack an overall strategy. Labour has access to well developed proposals for the reform of some aspects of health care, particularly community services like neighbourhood nursing, general practice and community care of the mentally ill.[8] Feminism has changed the perspectives of both NHS workers and users across a wide range of services, from midwifery to psychotherapy, and has produced a huge library of ideas and experiences from which the left can draw inspiration.[9] Health education is being shifted from a body of techniques designed to change the bad behaviour of individuals into a body of knowledge that can increase the power of individuals and groups to change their environments.[10] And we have the beginnings of a user-friendly slant to health policy in the renewal of the public health movement and the emergence of the Public Health Alliance.[11]

What the Labour Party lacks is a perspective on health economics and on the control of the health care machine. Without specific, workable ideas on health economics and NHS management, the left lacks credibility. For example, to say that this country is rich enough to afford the health service that it needs is acceptable to many socialists, but it is neither an argument nor a guide to action, but simply a truism. To urge something as grand as 'democracy' on the NHS and then descend into dull debates about the possible composition of Health Authorities is to evade the two central problems of NHS management. How to control the real consumers of health budgets, the professions linked closely to the drug and medical equipment industries in an increasingly integrated 'medical-industrial complex'? And how to make the individual citizen a genuine owner of the health service? Until political issues of that kind are addressed no amount of detailed planning of specific services will change the left's situation.

We should face reality. The strategy evolved by the labour movement for health care in the 1960s and 1970s has foundered, along with the political movements upon which it relied – powerful and militant trade unions, burgeoning local government and progressive professional ideologies. Unfortunately, old habits die hard. Even in Thatcher's third term too many act as if Thatcherism were simple interference in the left's political programme, and that normal politics will be resumed as soon as possible.[12] Progressive professionals busy dotting i's and crossing t's, and activists struggling for control of Labour's political machine have not noticed that someone has changed channels. We are left to guess what we are watching, and what it means.

Guessing is an uncomfortable business for a left built on certainties, but we have one consolation. The right has been guessing too, right up to 1988. The Conservatives have had no overriding game plan either, but have attacked issues aggressively, monitored reactions carefully and kept their options open. The demolition of the NHS has been prophesied for years, but has not yet occurred. The third term should offer Thatcher the chance to do away with the central institution of the Welfare State, but until the Prime

Minister announced a Cabinet review of ways of funding health care in response to the wave of protests in early 1988, no bold plan to replace the NHS with a system better suited to an enterprise culture had emerged. Even that unexpected and bellicose announcement did not mean that the Cabinet had such a plan, only that Margaret Thatcher felt that an opportunity to change the health service existed and that elements of a new approach were being assembled. The Carlton Club Conference of November 1987 may have been the intellectual turning point for the Conservatives, with its assembly of prominent figures from within the NHS and its detailed plans for a new kind of health service.[13] The government's inability to act decisively until now points to the difficulties that Conservatism has had in coping with health care politics. The high profile health service campaigns of the winter of 1987-88 underline Tory vulnerability, and will continue to give Labour a chance to push the government back onto the defensive as long as professional bodies, trade unions and user organisations can find and hold common ground.

Future Options

What are the possible outcomes of the present political crisis around the NHS? How long can the crisis continue, and who will resolve it? We do not know. Worse still, there is no imperative to find out, even as the Conservatives gather their ideas and strength to impose a market-oriented reform on the NHS. With so many trade unionists still arguing that there is nothing wrong with the health service that cannot be put right with extra money, the left has to make guessing do where informed debate would give better answers.

There is more at risk here than socialists' love of certainty. In the absence of a powerful critical tradition within health care we will be forced to think and act at a faster pace than usual, with less experience to go on, if the basis of the NHS is to be salvaged. Making sense of the bewildering events, actors and plots in the increasingly dramatic politics of health is difficult enough for the tiny minority close to the centre of activity. It is almost impossible for the majority who have no tradition of involvement in such politics.

Unable to work from existing ideas and concepts, we must improvise. With many possibilities for the development of the health service in front of us, we need to look at many options, not decide on some 'line' that of necessity would be arbitrary. One way to do that is guess at a few futures and see how they work. That way we can fit events into a series of pictures and by jumping ahead look back at how the critical period 1987-1990 might have been.

I have made up three histories from the larger number possible at the time of writing. They reflect my biases and contain all the flaws of futurology, but if we examine these three guesswork scenarios we can get some idea of the range of feasible political options open to the left. The first assumes that the Conservative counter-attack on funding, launched in the beginning of 1988, is effective in routing the government's critics. The second looks at a more finely balanced political settlement, and the third anticipates a powerful and durable political campaign led by the labour movement. All three scenarios move from the immediate past, the winter of 1987-88, to the point in the future where the Conservatives lose government office.

Scenario 1: 2012 – Picking up the Pieces

Margaret Thatcher's variant of Conservatism does not obey the rules learned by socialists educated in the political conflicts of the late 1960s and early 1970s. It does not bend, even under considerable pressure, and its resistance to change by external forces seems to have increased since the election victory of 1987. A huge majority in the House of Commons provides the bedrock of such intransigence, but there is more to Conservative determination than simple Parliamentary arithmetic.

The government can rely on differences amongst its opponents as well as its own influence and network of supporters within the health service to achieve its objectives. The progression of 'Hospital Alert' from a local campaign to a national protest organisation may have no measurable impact on government tactics except, perhaps, to encourage the Cabinet to accelerate its hastily constructed programme of changes. The trade union movement may well have the power to halt an unwanted reform of the NHS, but whether it will be able to use that power is another matter. On recent experience the necessary agreement around strategy may not be achieved and maintained, partly because it is very difficult to produce harmony within a federation of increasingly disparate unions which have a much looser commitment to the health service than political mythology suggests.

Even if agreement can be obtained, there is a substantial policy gap towards health care within the trade union movement. Most union members may think about the NHS in a relatively uncritical way, perhaps seeing its main problem as one of getting extra funding for new technology whose value is accepted unquestioningly, whilst unions like NUPE with a direct involvement in the service and an interface with professionalism take a more complex and appropriate view that is harder to reduce to attractive slogans.

There is also an enormous difference in the experience that trade unionists have of the health service, depending upon their age and where they live, but also on their occupation. The anger of nurses and other hospital workers about what is happening to them and to their work seems much greater now than it has been at any time since the pay dispute of 1982, but that feeling has not permeated the wider labour movement and does not shape the movement's agenda. Nurses already frustrated by the cautiousness of the Royal College of Nursing may want their resentments and fears expressed openly and forcibly by trade unions. Inevitably they feel let down if the labour movement's tone is too amiable, as happened at the rally at the end of the TUC demonstration for the NHS held on 5 March 1988 when nurses attempted to get onto a platform that represented a broader audience, but excluded them.

There is ample scope here for Conservative success by default. If, for example, the TUC does not respond to pressure from constituent unions and organise some kind of public activity around the time of the fortieth birthday of the NHS then individual unions will do so, perhaps without joint consultation and according to different perspectives, but with many opportunities for conflict and rivalry at local level. The obvious escape route for trade unions is to concentrate on the most pressing problems where the machinery for inter-union collaboration is established – privatisation and pay negotiation – and give secondary status to the wider issue of the health service's character.

Professional politics

Professional organisations seem to thrive under policies of 'divide and rule'. The government also has an important weapon within the medical profession in the Conservative Medical Association, which seems able to convey Conservative thinking directly to the decision-making levels of academic and clinical medicine, and to organise an important body of opinion that can advise government.

This potent combination of in-built insularity and an effective political network may be *the* factor that allows Thatcher's government to survive the immediate political crisis around the NHS. For example, there is likely to be pressure from general practitioners within the BMA for the leaders of that organisation to urge moderation on their hospital colleagues, for fear that the government would withdraw the favourable financial proposals within the Primary Care Bill. ('Good' practices look set to increase their incomes for only a little extra paperwork whilst 'bad' practices take a beating for their indifference.[14]) That message is being reinforced by periodic attacks by both Conservative backbenchers and Ministers on the medical profession's assumptions that it knows best for the nation's health, and in particular that the core group of clamorous specialists make good use of public resources. Public protest by surgeons and physicians can then be dismissed as 'shroud-waving', an unsavoury form of special pleading unconnected to overall public needs.

The same approach can be taken with independent academic reviews of NHS funding. Both the King's Fund Institute and the Institute of Health Service Management seem to be sensitive to government requirements, and it has been rumoured that within them views unfavourable to the Conservative perspective have escaped publicity because of the influence of government supporters. If that attempt at control fails, as seems likely at the time of writing, the intellectual climate will have altered in favour of increasing the amount of private provision in health care, and unrepentant authors of unfavourable judgements can be portrayed as examples of the very bad NHS management that Tories castigate so frequently.

The Royal College of Nursing may be less susceptible than the BMA to direct government influence, but it is no less insular. The more that the main issue for nurses can be presented as 'to strike or not to strike', the greater the Conservatives' advantage over the whole nursing profession. The RCN's existence depends on the distance it can put between itself and the rival trade unions, not simply because its membership is genteel (though some members are) but because it can represent one response to the ambivalence NHS workers feel towards industrial action. The rationale for the RCN would disappear if the trade unions recruiting nurses could incorporate that ambivalence and resolve it, but as yet they cannot, and they will not be given time to change by this government. The Conservatives will continue to emphasise the commitment of 'decent' NHS staff to their patients, and to hint at rewards for those who maintain this stance, so keeping the debate locked in terms favourable to themselves and to the RCN whilst allowing scope for political developments that would exclude the labour movement. Some kind of review of nursing, focussed on staffing levels, job descriptions and education – all issues on which the Royal College of Nursing has the advantage over its rivals – would reinforce the RCN argument that their isolation pays off for nurses.

The government will be encouraged by these signs of caution within the health service, and take the carefully maintained isolation of the professional organisations as a signal to refuse further concessions, beyond the one-off extra payment of £100 million and mortgage help for nurses anounced in autumn 1987.[15] To prevent any misinterpretation of this intransigence the Conservatives will continue to make reassuring gestures about their commitment to the health service, at least until the details of a reform package are worked out. For example, the Prime Minister will be able to restate her opposition to 'hotel charges' for hospital in-patients as evidence of government commitment to the principles of the NHS, without compromising future reform plans because such charges, whilst popular in the Tory backwoods, make little economic sense.

Bandwagons roll

The political tone will be set by the media attention given to assorted right-wing 'thinkers' with radical plans for restructuring health care. In the past leading Conservatives have been careful to keep such ideologues at a distance, using their proposals as possible strategic visions, and no more, but they now have other uses for the ultra-right. The appearance of advocates of extreme solutions, like the overnight abolition of the NHS in favour of entirely commercial health insurance, creates a political climate which the government can be seen to moderate by its own, less radical but no less substantial, reforms. Even before the Conservatives' own proposals reach daylight, core ideas from within their package can be floated and tried out. These advance warnings not only test opinion, but also help to make it.

For example, one-time Health Minister Gerard Vaughan, now an advisor to the private health insurance company Health First, has revealed that the government spent six years sitting on an internal DHSS report predicting an NHS cash crisis in 1987-88. He has urged the government to 'change the whole system', describing the NHS as 'extraordinarily wasteful, even after the administrative reforms of recent years', and to no one's surprise has advocated an insurance based system instead.[16] This looks like yet another rather cranky solution from an undistinguished Conservative politician, now on the sidelines, and perhaps that is what it was. But Dr Vaughan was also President of the Conservative Medical Society and a participant in the Carlton Club seminar that combined professional fire-power with detailed proposals for a fundamental restructuring of the NHS.

As well as manipulating the range of debate about NHS funding, the government will be able to take advantage of the attention given to more specific proposals for change emerging from the Warnock Committee's report on embryo research and the Griffiths report on the future organisation of Community Care services. At a time when all health workers might want to concentrate on the major political issue developing before their eyes, pressing problems of clinical care and everday work will crowd in and demand responses. Even when the main theme of the character of the NHS does become the central topic, powerful pressures will have skewed the terms of the debate. Health service staff will still polarise around the 'strike or not' dilemma whilst ward nurses worry so much about costs that campaigns to switch off lights in side-rooms may take precedence over consideration of funding principles.

Radical reform

That is the climate in which the Cabinet's own report will appear, causing more shock and anger than the March 1988 Budget's hand-outs to the rich. Taking their cue from the Carlton Club seminar, the government will use the health service's fortieth birthday as the opportunity to launch 'Basic Health Care', the newly reorganised National Health Service in which District Health Authorities will have financial responsibility for their services, using central government grants supplemented by local funding, and local hospitals will have the right to opt out of this DHSS-run franchise and find other financial backers. 'Basic Health Care' will be able to compete with commercial hospitals for insured patients, and the introduction of a state insurance system based on existing National Insurance payments will be scheduled for a date in the very near future.

The commercial medical sector will move on the back of this plan. American Medical International's UK-based operation has already become the first of the commercial medical organisations to be floated on the stock market, and other will follow it. Commercial investment in new hospital starts will rise rapidly, with US-based corporations leading the field, and private health insurance companies will continue to extend their benefits to include general practice and some types of 'alternative' medicine as well as clinical psychology, short-term psychotherapy, physiotherapy and midwifery.

Setting the tone

The events of 1988 will set the tone for health politics for a decade. In the next decade there will be a dramatic increase in the number of people enrolled in private health insurance, mostly through deals made by their employers, with perhaps a third or more of the population in private schemes. Dual services will operate for insured and 'Basic Health Care' patients from the same sites, particularly in general practice but also in some 'BHC' hospitals. Charges will be introduced for NHS preventive care, including contraception, which has been a free service since 1974. The network of registered 'alternative' practitioners will double to nearly 16,000 and a new professional organisation may form, the British Alternative Medicine Association, perhaps with its launch conference sponsored by two health insurance companies and a major 'health food' concern.

This diversification of funding sources and the differential growth of commercial hospitals in different areas will increase the variability of services across the country. The public system will stay dominant but of course remain underfunded in the poorer Health Regions of the North, Scotland and South Wales. Commercial medicine will dominate in the South-East and expand to rival but not overtake the public service in the South-West, the Midlands and East Anglia.

The downturn
This evolution of a multi-tier system will stop because the Conservative economic boom of the mid- to late 1980s will peter out, particularly in the North but also in the Tory heartlands of the South. Inflationary pressures will prompt the return of wage militancy, which will affect the commercial medical sector in ways previously not seen. Slow-down in economic growth will reduce the personal disposable income of the moderately affluent and make them think twice about private health insurance, even when offered as a fringe benefit in lieu of salary rises. Increases in health insurance premiums will reinforce the slow but measurable decline of the insurance sector, and the quality of 'Basic Health Care' services will regain the attention of the educated and affluent.

At some point in the 1990s market fluctuations and investment decisions made by transnational corporations with headquarters outside the UK will make the commercial medical sector unstable and a source of recurrent scandals. Media reports will highlight the over-investigation of ill people by commercial clinics keen to enlarge medical bills, and the rising operation rates for minor problems that could have been dealt with in less expensive and traumatic ways. Instances of poor treatment where money, not professional judgement, motivated the practitioners will make harrowing television documentaries. The shoddy care of elderly infirm men and women 'warehoused' by commercial nursing homes will alarm the insured middle-aged, who have become an increasingly powerful group in an ageing society.

Public pressure for the introduction of new services based on new technology will continue to grow, fuelled by the 'greying' of the population and by the marketing methods of high-tech companies desperate to regain the vast sums spent on research. Pressure to introduce a nationwide screening programme to identify and treat people who have biochemical predictors for cancer of the breast, bowel and stomach in their bloodstream will cause fright in the Treasury and in transnational corporations alike because accountants forecast that the launch, follow-up and treatment costs of the cancer prediction and treatment programme will equal a quarter of the then current 'Basic Health Care' bill. Anxiety about this programme will be amplified as the death toll from cervical cancer rises above 3,000 per year. The majority of the activists in the campaigns for wide-scale cancer screening come from the generation of women who became sexually active during the late 1960s and early 1970s, and who are now entering the high-risk age range for a disease that could have been detected early, had the money to develop and maintain public screening services not dried up in the 1990s.

Anxious for new sources of money, smarting from public criticism and keen for firm guidance, Britain's poorly co-ordinated medical services, reminiscent of those of the period between the First and Second World Wars, will be integrated under local authority control and central government financing by a reforming administration that introduces a redistributive taxation system, abolishes compulsory retirement, legislates for a twenty-hour working week and embarks on a programme of re-industrialisation to revive a stagnant economy, reduce unemployment and renew welfare and health services. The question is, when?

The Conservatives are likely to win a fourth term, even if

the economic downturn begins to bite in the South before 1992. The Tory majority is so large, and the electoral system so undemocratic, that the political consequences of further deterioration in the balance of payments, continued decline in the Northern economy and overheating in the South will take much longer to work through the system. A dramatic external event, comparable in scale with the Falklands War, might break the Conservatives' grip, as might an unexpected political outburst comparable to the French 'May Events' of 1968, but it would be unwise to make these outside possibilities the centre-piece of a socialist strategy.

If the opposition remains as divided and uninspiring as it is at the moment, Thatcherism might have a fifth term and lead us into a period of centre-left coalition politics in the first decade of the twenty-first century. We have no reason to believe that a mass conversion to socialism (in any form) will occur once the Conservatives fail, particularly since Thatcherism will have redefined the nature of education, housing, transport, urban living, trade unionism, welfare services and health care. The end of a phase of political compromise between the centre-right and the centre-left may take almost as long as the end of Thatcherism itself. In this pessimistic scenario a left-wing government as radical as Thatcher's may not appear until the beginning of the second decade of the third millenium.

Scenario 2: 1996 – The Pendulum Swings

Whilst the potential for conflict and division amongst the government's enemies is very great, public enthusiasm for the NHS is greater. That deep-rooted commitment may be enough to overcome the apparently congenital sectarianism of the left and impose a political solution to the crisis of health care that is neither Thatcherite nor mainstream socialist.

Despite the government's counter-propaganda, and intense lobbying within the medical profession by the Conservative Medical Society, the 'Hospital Alert' campaign was able to recapture media attention early in 1988 with plans for a lobby of parliament on 25 February, contributing to the high profile given to the plight of the health service in the weeks prior to the protest. The lobby was large but less representative of the areas of the country in which the NHS was most threatened by cuts than hoped for by its organisers. This caused some campaigners to suspect that parts of the middle classes whose involvement in defence of the NHS was so much sought had already given up and gone over to private provision, but that was not the only explanation.

'Hospital Alert' was a new organisation, operating on a shoestring, a little too middle-class to recruit trade union involvement easily, proposing an action that may have seemed of limited value against a government proud of its deafness. In the circumstances the lobby might be judged a success, a contributor to the backdrop of public protest in the run-up to the TUC-sponsored demonstrations in major centres on 5 March 1988. These were hugely succesful in terms of labour movement involvement, although the press and television minimised their coverage in news reporting. Approaching 100,000 people paraded past Downing Street, 10,000 marched in Scottish Health Minister Michael Forsyth's Stirling constituency and five columns converged from Birmingham's main general hospitals to a rally in the central Chamberlain Square.

The persistence of public protest about the state of the NHS meant that official claims that the health service was booming and blooming began to backfire on the DHSS and on the increasingly disliked Health Ministers, Tony Newton and Edwina Currie. The mood of the country is such that a series of well publicised scandals, including the avoidable death of a baby girl in an inadequately staffed neonatal unit, reduce government popularity and threaten the Conservatives' poll lead over Labour. Junior Minister Currie, speaking at a meeting in Southampton, makes the situation worse by saying that:

> People with cash to spare might consider postponing a second holiday and using the money for a non-urgent operation. They might put off decorating the living room and get their teeth done instead.

This child-like remark is a gift to the opposition, as Labour MPs point out that 40 per cent of the population had no holiday at all in 1986, according to government statistics, and that the great majority of people were increasingly anxious about having to choose between a first holiday and an essential operation.[17]

Heavyweight criticism

Own goals of this kind are insufficient even to embarrass Thatcherites, but the spread of criticism from the natural opponents of Conservatism to within its own ranks creates a much greater threat. The House of Commons Social Services Select Committee, with an in-built Conservative majority, calls on the government to fund all NHS pay awards in full, to provide an extra £1.1 billion to compensate for expected 1987-88 shortfall of £95 million and to find the £1 billion judged necessary to restore clinical services.[18]

Within days of publication of the Select Committee report the British Medical Association publishes a survey of 'acute' hospital services which shows that the NHS had lost 3,940 beds in 1987, mostly because of cash shortages, and highlights the widespread cancellations of out-patient and operating theatre sessions because of staff shortages. Arguing for a cash injection of £300 million and full payment of pay awards, the BMA also proposes investment of between £500,000 and £1 million over three to five years to develop the necessary information technology to facilitate resource management.[19]

Under increasing pressure from within her party, and aware that the reports on health care funding soon to appear from the IHSM and the King's Fund Institute are likely to argue for the status quo and more resources despite the efforts of government supporters within the commissions, the Prime Minister announces a Cabinet enquiry into NHS funding. In effect the Conservatives accept the arguments for extra funding, but attempt to shift the debate from the amount needed to its source, all the while arguing that the public purse can give no more. This produces apprehension within the opposition, which had not expected such a move and which saw the Carlton Club seminar's arguments as the Cabinet's blueprint for a market-oriented health service.

This overestimates the radicalism of the government, which has been unable to assault the NHS directly in its previous two terms and which remains unsure about the extent and depth of potential resistance to any attempt to impose radical changes in health care. Even though the professional, consumer and trade union opposition remains unco-ordinated and divided, its apparent strength is sufficient to make the Conservatives cautious. The Cabinet's report draws back from the option of dismantling the NHS, promising instead the introduction of tax relief on private health insurance premiums and hinting at legislation to permit general practitioners and others to found commercial 'health shops' in which professionals of different disciplines could combine. The Conservatives survive Budget Day in 1988 without conceding extra money for the health service, even though public opinion favours a cash boost to the NHS in preference to tax cuts.[20]

Autumn heat

1988 is the critical year for the NHS. In it the professional organisations combine to launch joint campaigns calling for an increase in public spending on health care, using the every-day contact health service staff have with the public as the distribution mechanism for their appeal for support. The campaigns aim to turn 'middle England' against the Prime Minister, who will make the mistake of defending her beleaguered Health Ministers too often and too stridently. To an extent they succeed, although this is will not be apparent at the time since no major change in government policy occurs.

Trade unions inside and outside the NHS will join these campaigns, though not without some petulant grassroots criticism of the 'johnny-come-lately' style of the professional bodies. No official collaboration between trade unions and the BMA or RCN occurs, despite background contact, and there will be no doubt that the professional organisations are the dominant partner in the protest movement. For all the criticism from trade union activists, the secondary position of the labour movement will be tolerated by the mass of union members.

This shift of gear by health service workers could be enough to change the political climate. Once again critical voices will greet government Ministers wherever they try to argue their case, and although the language of confrontation used by professionals may be less inflammatory and less intimidatory than many socialists might like, it will become effective. A critical mass of informed opinion will make dissent normal and acceptable, and make official orthodoxy look foolish and ill considered. For the first time since Falklands jingoism coincided with the beginnings of the consumer boom in 1983, Conservative voters will keep quiet about their allegiance.

With support slipping away, and the economy in the South overheating with continued house-price inflation and the beginnings of a wages offensive by organised workers, the Thatcher government may need to buy back public approval. One way of regaining credit would be to introduce new money into the NHS, not in a quantity that would appear as a sign of weakness before protest, but perhaps proportionate to recent increases in consumer purchasing power. Unpopular Ministers could be transfered away from the DHSS in a Cabinet reshuffle, and a whispering campaign to blame recent political problems on their incompetence would be easy to encourage in a still servile press.

This would be a change in policy, but less than a U-turn. The NHS would still not be safe in Conservative hands, and the process of change would have been slowed but not necessarily diverted. Much would then depend on the responses of the dominant and subordinate components of the protest wave. If professional, consumer and trade union organisations respond in harmony, perhaps welcoming the new funding as evidence of the government's conversion to good sense, but also firmly pointing out that it will only buy a short-term reprieve, the Conservatives may not regain their earlier initiative. Debates about the future of the health service that can be shaped, at least in part, by the agenda of the labour movement will then become important, as ideas about health care that do not rely upon market forces as their driving force are sought.

As this political shift coincides with a slow-down in the growth rate of the economy, the expansion of commercial medicine will halt, and perhaps begin to reverse. Recruitment to private health insurance programmes will decline, causing the insurance companies considerable problems. The earlier influx of the newly insured will have increased claims against health insurance as enthusiastic subscribers hurry to try out their new privileges. A decline in recruitment may mean a cash-flow crisis, with reserves being used to bridge the gap between diminishing premiums and increasing claims. Increases in premiums and reductions in benefits would follow, and the decline in profits might be enough to provoke US-based investors in commercial medicine to sell off their UK assets.

Goodbye, Prime Minister
The scene will be set for a dramatic change – the resignation of the Prime Minister. This may seem surprising and unlikely, but it would be a wise move for Margaret Thatcher and for the Conservative Party. Economic growth is unlikely to stay on target, the stock market crash of 1987 having soured UK investment more than the government expected. Unemployment will probably rise again, despite continued manipulation of the figures. Once the press discovers the astonishing growth in the number of people on long-term sickness benefit – switched away from the unemployment queues but capable of working if there had been jobs to do – an ugly scandal will evolve. Kenneth Baker's Education Act will become the focus of intense discontent, and campaigns against the poll tax will make inroads into Conservative support, particularly in the South-East. By then Mrs Thatcher will be tired and apprehensive, and will hand over before her still considerable personal popularity wanes further.

The Conservative Party will still have the flexibility to produce a successor. The succession will be smooth, as will the new leader. An image of moderation, not intransigence, will be projected from Downing Street. The media spotlight will move away from the NHS even though Health Authorities and professional organisations continue to warn that the problem of underfunding has not been solved. An early election might be used as a way of avoiding some major embarrassment over the NHS, perhaps from an imminent government-sponsored report that will document the shoddy state of health service buildings, or before the BMA can ballot for industrial action when the Doctors Pay Review Body recommendations are ignored yet again.

The Conservatives will win that early General Election,

but with the party's majority greatly reduced. Rising unemployment is likely to be the key issue that swings voters towards the centre parties, with worry about the state of the health service a secondary concern. Consumer organisations of the 'Hospital Alert' kind will reform, highlighting the predicted return of a funding crisis in the NHS. Some chance event may upset all the political calculations – maybe a catastrophic fire in one of the 'tower block' hospitals built in the late 1960s, which shocks the country. *Guardian* political commentators will begin to speculate on the return of a Labour government at the next election, scheduled for 1996.

Scenario 3: 1992 – Thatcher's Waterloo

Even at this late stage, the political crisis around the NHS could destroy the Thatcher government. The entry of the BMA and the Royal College of Nursing into the campaign for greater health service spending has already galvanised the trade unions. A series of 'days of action' resulted in large demonstrations in every major city, huge lobbies of parliament and – unexpectedly – sporadic industrial action. Although the government refused to provide extra NHS funding before the March 1988 Budget, the opportunity still exists for creative accountants within the DHSS to give some covert financial help to the hardest hit Health Regions, perhaps by writing off some overspending. This small signal of Conservative nervousness might not convince the opposition that an all-out attack on Thatcher's government would succeed, but the Tories might just come to the left's aid.

Not only are some Ministers own-goal artists, but Thatcherite Conservatism has a crude political style that can be counter-productive. It might only need a clumsy Tebbit-style attempt by government Ministers to censor television news and documentaries on the health service to fuel the protests. Government action against illegal industrial action might spark off more strikes as industrial workers feel doubly assaulted, through the erosion of their rights and of their health service. Failure to act against illegal industrial action, or use of nominally independent anti-union groups to initiate legal action against strikers, might appear as further evidence of Conservative weakness. A nightmare scenario then unfolds for the Conservatives, with no escape from political conflict available to their government.

By then the unpredictability of health service politics will have confounded the pessimists who had waved goodbye to the NHS earlier in the year. Militancy amongst nurses will increase as protest grows, and although the RCN membership will continue to uphold its 'no strike' policy, local collaboration between RCN and TUC-affiliated unions will produce spectacular and imaginative protest actions across the country, as it did in the earlier part of 1988. This upsurge in campaigning will renew contacts between workers in different industries and from different backgrounds, reviving local trade union and community spirit and organisation and prompting a renaissance of grassroots activity.

The role of the labour movement will be crucial to defeating the government. A major TUC initiative, perhaps focussed on the fortieth birthday of the Health Service in July 1988, could become the launching pad for a frontal attack on the government. This would mean a qualitative change in the attitude and activity of the TUC, and some innovative approaches to suspicious professionals and an anxious public, but such changes are possible, especially in the critical situation created by the Conservatives. Thatcher's aggressive response to the protests of 1987-88, with acceleration of plans for NHS reform, took the left and the trade unions by surprise, but it need not disarm them and prevent an equal and opposite reaction.

Tactical withdrawal
We may be so mesmerised by the intransigence of Thatcherism that we cannot see that, at least for the NHS, it is more style than substance. The threat of a major political confrontation, perhaps on the scale of the miners' strike but over a bigger and more popular industry, may be enough for new realism to break out within the Conservative government. Inside the Cabinet the arguments of DHSS Ministers will overcome the Treasury's insistence that no further public spending is possible. Education Ministers will support their DHSS colleagues,

noting that the hostility to Baker's Bill had increased rather than decreased during recent months as protestors grew confident and saw through the government's facade of strength. Civil servants responsible for planning the transition from local rates to the poll tax are likely to play an important part in nuturing new realism, pointing out the risks of defying public opinion on several issues simultaneously, and commenting on the unease of Tory back-benchers with Home Counties seats troubled by grassroots campaigns against the tax.

The Prime Minister will have few options left, and extra funding for the NHS, including a special fund to provide extra services for AIDS sufferers and a commitment to find extra cash to meet nurses' pay rises in full, would be one of them. Once again, the responses of the professional, consumer and trade union organisations will determine the next phase of events. If a broad front of agreement is not maintained, or the agreement is too lenient on the government, the Conservatives will gain time to reorganise and counter-attack. The money cannot be refused, nor can it be accepted as the desired solution, since it will almost certainly fall far short of the realistic figure needed to restore lost services and renew NHS growth. At the same time a protest movement of such heterogeneous composition will not survive a move to topple the government itself, and the pressures from within the trade union movement and the left to seek that outcome would have to resisted.

That does not mean that the government will survive the conflict. As the protest movement grows and begins to alter Conservative policy, the stability of Thatcherism must diminish, and the number of different pressures on it will increase. Unpredictable events may become politically significant. Perhaps all the Health Ministers will be replaced in a 'Night of the Long Scalpels' Cabinet reshuffle after an unexpectedly large demonstration in defence of the NHS halts London for a day. An apparently off-the-cuff remark about the obvious need for extra funding for the NHS made by Prince Charles at a City banquet in December will cause the Cabinet great embarrassment and shake party morale.

Faction fighting

This would be a good time for the Prime Minister to resign,

helped by discontent within the Conservative Party, to make way for a leader with a more moderate style. In the changed political environment her departure, and the growing 'wetness' of the party as a whole, might be enough to trigger an intense internal conflict, with the ultra-right denouncing centrists in an unprecedented display of factionalism. Once out in the open such a leadership struggle could last months, not days, adding to the unease at the sluggishness of the post-crash economy and pushing the government's popularity to still lower depths.

This bracing political climate succeeds where Neil Kinnock and his team had failed, reviving the Labour Party, which launches a campaign for 'A New Health Service', with four central policies:

> to increase spending on the NHS from just under 6 per cent of gross national product to the EEC average of 8 per cent over a five year period;

> to channel resources to points as close as possible to the citizen, at worksite, school and home ('Goodbye to the hospitals' says one glitzy Labour television commercial);

> to introduce a 'Bill of Patient's Rights' guaranteeing a specified range of health services to every UK resident;

> and to give every citizen his or her own medical record, encoded on a smart card, starting with the children born in the year 2000.

Against all the odds, the Conservative Party will lose the 1992 General Election. Although Labour will not win it, it must become the dominant partner in the hastily formed coalition between Labour and the Social and Liberal Democrats. (Dr David Owen, the only SDP member elected, will not be invited to join the coalition.)

Wishful Thinking

The first scenario is the most likely. It incorporates all the key elements we can identify in the present situation and the recent past: professional militancy combined with isolationism; government intransigence and a growing taste for both change and revenge; slow and incomplete responses from the labour movement; passivity from the bulk of the population, which observes events from the sidelines.

The second scenario may well be the hope of the more benign thinkers within the professions and perhaps within the left as well. It proves that orderly resistance to bad government does work, even against headstrong and victorious Conservatives. And the end result is that most desirable of things, a satisfying compromise. As an outcome it would be very much better than the first scenario, but it has an unrealistic feel to it, and it also has no conclusion. Would the new government survive, and if it did, would it be competent?

Most socialists would like the third scenario to come about. It would vindicate a strategy that was once sound, the alliance of a broad range of political opinions against an increasingly isolated enemy, and bring about an objective that is hopeful, the election of a Labour government with a progressive policy for health. Unfortunately it is the least likely outcome, for a number of reasons. Professional organisations are poor leaders of movements that topple Conservative governments. They are themselves over-commited to market solutions for health care problems, and their professionalism is founded upon a deep distrust of collectivist approaches to social welfare. The medical profession's reliance upon the pharmaceutical industry for education and research opportunities creates a real dependence that will be hard to break. The profession's preoccupation with money makes commercial medicine very attractive to some doctors, particularly in the South, so that the political climate encouraged a small proportion to jump the gun and 'go private' completely even though the majority of the profession stay with the bigger spender, the NHS.

The continued commitment of professionals to the fundamental idea of a centrally funded, comprehensive service free at the time of need cannot be taken for granted, even after the prominent and progressive role played by the British Medical Association and Royal College of Nursing in resistance to NHS cuts, because professionalism as an ideology and as social practice rests upon relationships between individual providers and individual users – the consultation, or the nursing tasks – which easily convert into trading relationships. The National Health Service has had an enormous impact on professional ideology, yet forty years of practicing medicine without taking money off ill people has not extinguished wallet-consciousness amongst hospital specialists, as the growth of commercial medicine demonstrates. And the pre-eminent representative body of nurses, the RCN, has learnt that there are political possibilities if not secure financial gains to be made from subordinating nurses' interests to the real or invented interests of a host of individual patients. Nursing has been made into a 'vocation', a form of easily exploited, one-sided giving that has used up the energy and devotion of huge numbers of women over the lifetime of the NHS.

In practice the professional organisations are likely to assert their very real differences with TUC-affiliated unions, even as they look for common ground for joint action. So they should, but the independence that they value most is freedom from labour, not from capital. Whilst the NHS remains the dominant source of jobs, resources and income, the professional bodies will defend it. Should its level of funding drop below a critical threshold, its credibility diminish and the commercial hospital network become a serious rival to public health services, then the professional thing to do will be to safeguard professional interests and look for alternative sources of finance. 'The public interest' will be invoked to justify the change, but only because professionals traditionally assume that what is good for the doctor or for the nurse is also good for their patients.

This shift of allegiance is less likely to happen if the trade union movement exerts enough pressure to unsettle the government and retain sufficient public backing for the existing arrangements. But can the labour movement achieve that? Trade unions may well campaign for the health service, but the political and economic climate is oppressive and discourages the kind of sanction – loss of industrial production – that might impress a government as determined, aggressive and competent as Thatcher's third administration. Sanctions may be most easily applied in service industries in which workers identify closely with the NHS, but the services affected are likely to be most used by those with the greatest need for them, and for the NHS as well. A bus drivers' strike does not keep many BUPA subscribers shivering at bus stops. A power blackout in the City of London might carry the message to the most relevant social groups, but who will organise it?

This does not mean that a vigorous labour movement initiative on health policy is not worth pursuing. On the contrary, no other part of society is likely to be able to sustain long-term action for the NHS. Yet to become first amongst equals in an alliance with professional organisations that have strong feelings of class, occupational and moral superiority over trade unions would demand from the labour movement something it lacks – a strategy for changing the health service that would benefit both those who work in it and the great majority of those who currently use it.

Whilst the Labour Party has had energetic front bench health teams it lacks the policy-making apparatus to produce new ideas, the political machinery to educate its own supporters in those new ideas and to implement new policies, and even the political culture to promote medium-term campaigning work by its local branches. The normal political reflexes of the left move resolutions through committees, votes through meetings and people up and down administrative and career ladders, but they are poor responses to a government aiming for major social change. Hyperactive sectarians apart, most socialists have learned to think of politics only as a form of plodding, not running. The Conservatives are more athletic, and seem both psychologically and physically better prepared to sprint when the opportunity arises.

Can these deficiencies be put right in five years? Labour's election programme for the NHS in 1987 was not wrong in policy terms, but it was unimpressive in political terms, for it offered little guide to action for health workers or the public, and presented a vision of a worthy, well scrubbed future healthiness that correlated poorly with everday life. And whilst that could be put right, in a formal sense, with better packaging and presentation of policy, how can the left hope to initiate change if it cannot even identify labour movement activists and supporters within the NHS?

The Importance of Change

Our health service's history of underfunding, poorly paid staff, deteriorating building stock and rising usage will not go away. Labour does not yet have the solutions to these problems, although it might acquire them quickly once in office, beginning with overdue lessons in health economics and health service management. If Labour forms or dominates the nation's government after 1992, it will be in the same position as Thatcher's administration in its first two terms, forced to cobble together an approach towards health care, one hopes feeling its way from success to success, with the DHSS competing with other Ministries for Treasury attention. That would not be so bad, if only because it might encourage experimentation and a touch of pluralism in the new government's approach to health care, but it would also be a risky situation. Plodders can make good experimenters, given time, but the pressures that confront Thatcher's Health Ministers and that are described in the rest of this book, would still impinge on government and demand rapid solutions.

Nevertheless, the chance of government office would be a fine thing, and we should not miss opportunities to block Conservative advances and, perhaps, push them onto the defensive. Every campaign against local cuts does matter, however hopeless it may seem at the time, because it harasses a much larger and more powerful enemy. Every delay and failure to provide services needs publicity, just as every success by NHS staff working against the odds needs praise. Yet even on this familiar ground we cannot take too much for granted. Much that was solid has already melted into air. By capturing the political agenda Conservatism has converted progressive ideas into instruments in the market's hidden hand. 'Care in the community' has become a cost-cutting exercise that releases real estate almost as fast as it releases mentally ill people from inadequate but at least existing care. 'Prevention' and 'health promotion' have been filleted of their meaning and turned into marketable and potentially chargeable commodities in a society in which health hazards are accumulating fast. Planning has become a device for anticipating and costing throughput, rather than a tool for measuring outcomes and needs. Much of the left's intellectual capital has been stolen, and more must be accumulated.

This may seem pessimistic, but only if we view possibilities in terms carried over from the 1970s. Margaret Thatcher's swift adoption of alternative funding sources as the main political issue of 1988 shows that sudden changes are possible, and we should be on the look-out for their early signs, without making the third scenario our only hope in the way that Labour in local government banked on a Kinnock victory in 1987. Preparation for either of the first two scenarios is necessary because they are more realistic, and it may even be a precondition for success if scenario three works out after all. The more thought now put into the politics of professionalism, the problems of funding and the impact of new technology, the better the left will deal with those issues with or without electoral success. The rest of this book is a tentative attempt at such preparation.

Notes and References

1 Richard Piauchaud, 'The Growth of Poverty', in *The Growing Divide: A Social Audit, 1979-1987*, editors Carol Walker and Alan Walker, Child Poverty Action Group publication no. 72, 1987, pp.22-3.

2 M.E.J. Wadsworth, 'Serious Illness in Childhood and its Association with Later Life Achievement', in *Class and Health: Research and Longitudinal Data*, editor Richard Wilkinson, Tavistock, 1986.

3 See Hilary Graham and Margaret Stacey, 'Socio-economic Factors Related to Child Health' in *Progress in Child Health*, Vol. 1, editor J.A. Macfarlane, Churchill Livingstone, 1984.

4 In October 1987 threats of legal action by an individual refused kidney dialysis by Central Birmingham Health Authority brought a speedy cash injection from Health Minister Tony Newton. A month later a second attempt at using the courts to force the same Health Authority to treat the baby boy needing cardiac surgery failed. ('Is There a Solicitor in the House?', *Health Services Journal*, 26 November 1987)

5 A study from Leicestershire showed that 49 per cent of in-patients were readmitted with the same complaint fewer than 30 days after a previous admission. (James Jones, 'The Price of Early Discharge', *Health Services Journal*, 19 June 1986)

6 A marked downturn in spending on priority client groups in the community by London Health Authorities between 1976 and 1984 has meant that in the capital the numbers of psychiatric inpatients has decreased but that anticipated community services have not developed. (*Losing Patients: A Report on the Position of Priority Groups in London*, Greater London Association of Community Health Councils, 1987)

7 In the autumn of 1987 the National Association of Health Authorities (NAHA) called for an 8.3 per cent increase in the NHS budget, to bring it to a total of £12.2 billion, but this money was not forthcoming from the government. A

report produced jointly by the Institute of Health Service Managers (IHSM), the British Medical Association and the Royal College of Nursing advocating that NHS funding should rise in line with national income was dismissed as having a 'superficially attractive simplicity' by Health Minister Tony Newton. IHSM President Barbara Young called for London Health Authorities to collaborate to prevent ad hoc cuts packages from creating 'black spots' where services would fall below adequate levels. She cited the situation that had developed when one third of the city's neurosurgery beds had been closed simultaneously without Health Authorities being aware of what was happening. (*Health Services Journal*, 22 October 1987)

8 See, as examples: *Neighbourhood Nursing – A Focus for Care* (the Cumberledge Report), HMSO, 1986; *The Future Organisation of Primary Medical Care*, Medical Practitioners Union, 1986, and the work which inspired the MPU's policy, Julian Tudor Hart, 'A New Kind of Family Doctor', *Socialism and Health*, January-February 1986.

9 The impact of the women's movement on health politics needs its own book, and the bibliography of political writing on health issues from feminist perspectives is much greater than work done from within the socialist tradition. A taste of this can be had from *Feminist Practices in Women's Health Care*, editor Christine Webb, John Wiley & Sons, 1986.

10 As examples of this change, see *The Politics of Health Education: Raising the Issues*, editors Sue Rodmell and Alison Watt, Routledge & Kegan Paul, 1986 and Jeff French and Lee Adams, 'From Analysis to Synthesis: Theories of Health Education', *Health Education Journal*, 1986, 45, 2, pp.71-3.

11 See Shirley Goodwin, 'The Public Health Alliance', *Medicine in Society*, 1987, 13, 2, pp.15-7.

12 The sudden outbreak of anger and action amongst nurses, starting with a local protest in Manchester but rapidly spreading to involve health service workers in many parts of the country, rejuvenated those parts of the left that recognise only industrial action as genuine politics. The revival was temporary, since the government needed only to weather the protests and hold to its Budget plans to cut taxes and freeze NHS spending for the hyperactivist phase to pass. And pass it did, losing momentum as its limited impact was noted. We overestimate the nature of the political understanding of the majority of those who work in or use the NHS, and who are prepared to act in its defence. Far from being to the left of the political machine, that majority is to the right, with the nurses' campaign arising from an amalgam of national and local issues and general and specific grievances. In Scotland privatisation was an important issue, in Manchester threats to withdraw special duty payments sparked a response, and in London weighting was an issue. Add to those grievances the consistent refusal on the part of the government to abide by the recommendations of the nurses independent pay review body established by the Conservatives as a reward for the RCN's 'no strike' policy, and stir in the rivalry between the RCN, NUPE and COHSE, and a potent recipe for conflict appears. The expression of anger by nurses is not the only novel feature of this weak and unfocussed dispute; the new reality of trade unions under Thatcher asserted itself, with division amongst unionists between those who favour a cautious and limited defence of their members' interests and those who opt to defy a bad government. (Jolyon Jenkins, 'Will the Nurses Beat the Thatcher Review?', *New Statesman*, 29 January 1988)

13 This is not an attempt to disguise the undercurrent of hostility towards the NHS that has existed within the Conservative Party since the 1940s, but a corrective to the widespread conspiracy theory that substitutes for understanding and examination on the left. Ideas about how the NHS should be dismantled or modified out of recognition have a long pedigree in the Tory Party, as documented by Herman Grunwald in 'The Tories' Love for the NHS',

Medicine in Society, 1983, 9, 1, pp.22-5, but they have been minority views that have failed to dent mainstream Conservative commitment to the post-war consensus on the welfare state. Even after 1979, with the growth of a far-right 'think-tank' industry the advocates of insurance systems, vouchers and health maintainance organisations have been kept at arm's length and used as sources of long-term perspective, not short-term tactics and medium-term strategy. If that situation has changed, the change has occurred recently, most probably in the autumn of 1987 with the 'experts meeting' convened jointly by the Carlton Club and the Conservative Medical Society. Amongst the conclusions of that meeting were proposals that have direct bearing on the fortieth birthday of the NHS, including:

> Retitling the NHS to show that its first forty years was the 'end of the beginning' and that, from 1988 onwards, a whole new concept of funding and services will take us into the twenty-first century;
> establishing the NHS as an independent statutory body with financial accountability, and moving from a centralised to a decentralised service;
> increasing the use of joint ventures between the NHS and the private sector, creating an integrated and interrelated market;
> extending the principles of charging and creating a costed service;
> creating, in conjunction with the private sector, a National Health Insurance Scheme, capitalising upon the new financial accountability of the service, to provide a health care plan for the nation;
> devolving all health care responsibility to directly funded District Health Authorities, and dismantling Regional Health Authorities. In this context individual hospitals could 'opt out', thereby instilling into the system a competitive element.

If there is a Conservative grand plan, this is likely to be it. (*The NHS and the Private Sector*, confidential proceedings of the Carlton Club meeting held in conjunction with the Conservative Medical Society, 30 November 1987)

14 The White Paper on Primary Care proposed, amongst other changes: financial incentives for doctors to provide health checks, to increase vaccinations, and to care for the elderly; new allowances for GPs who undertake education throughout their careers; a major role in child health surveillance (almost certainly with extra fees as reward); retirement at 70; reimbursement for a greater range and number of practice staff than currently permitted (two whole time equivalents per GP, working as nurse, receptionist/filing clerk, manager or computer operator. (*Promoting Better Health*, HMSO, 1987)

15 The mortgage help for nurses in the London area got off to a very poor start. Administered by the Nationwide Anglia Building Society, which aimed to offer 100 per cent mortages at values of 4.5 times personal income with an interest rate set at two-thirds of the normal, the scheme attracted only 600 applicants by mid-March 1988 instead of the anticipated 5,000. About half of these were joint applicants, for whom the scheme's viability was threatened by planned changes in mortgage tax relief in the March budget. The scheme was shelved until after the Budget, and the RCN described it as 'another gimmick'. (*Guardian*, 12 March 1988)

16 Despite the accumulated evidence that central funding and administration is cheaper and more efficient than commercial alternatives, and that sick people make poor shoppers, the erstwhile Health Minister insisted that an insurance system would be better than the NHS because it would give both users and providers an idea of treatment costs. (*Medical Monitor*, 11 January 1988)

17 Only one in five can afford two holidays a year, and the growth of DIY retailing suggests that few spend the price of dental care on getting in a painter and decorator. ('Currie's Cure', *New Society*, 5 February 1988)

18 The Select Committee's report made four key recommendations: the government should fund all the 1988-89 pay awards in full; enough money should be allocated in 1988-89 to allow 2 per cent service development; the government should make good the £95 million shortfall for 1987-88 immediately, and set aside at least £1 billion over the next two years for identified and costed measures 'to bring the NHS back up to scratch and restore the morale of its staff'; develop better ways of measuring effectiveness as a matter of urgency. ('A Touch of Sanity', *Health Service Journal*, 3 March 1988)

19 *The Crisis in the Acute Hospital Sector*, British Medical Association, 1988.

20 A Marplan poll conducted for the *Guardian* and published on the eve of the Budget gave the following percentage results:

Voting intention				Social class			
All	Cons	Lab	SLD/SDP	AB	C1	C2	D

Cut the standard rate of income tax by 1p?

9	19	4	3	13	12	9	5

Or spend the £1.2 billion it would cost on the NHS?

84	73	93	92	77	84	84	89

Cut the standard rate of income tax by 2p?

6	13	2	5	13	8	4	4

Or spend the £2.4 billion it would cost on the NHS?

62	47	74	64	52	61	60	69

(*Guardian*, 14 March 1988)

A Marplan poll commissioned jointly by *Health Services Journal* and the National Association of Health Authorities, and published in April 1987, showed somewhat lower levels of support for increasing NHS income from taxation compared with the 1988 responses, although the questions were different and the 1988 respondents were considering foregoing a planned tax cut rather than increasing taxation.

'From which source should extra finance be raised?'

	Class			
	ABC1		C2DE	
Government expenditure	41	(46)	48	(49)
Increase prescription charges	1	(4)	2	(1)
Contribution by patients to treatment cost	15	(15)	10	(11)
Increased taxation	21	(15)	21	(11)

The figures in brackets refer to answers given to the same questions in 1985, and show an increase in the percentages of respondents wanting taxation increased to fund the NHS. (Peter Davies, 'The Public Voices its Opinions on the NHS', *Health Services Journal*, 2 April 1987, pp.382-3)

2 The Erosion of Principles

The principles upon which the National Health Service was founded no longer apply. Successive governments of both parties have modified a medical service that was intended to be free at the time of need, comprehensive in scope and financed by the Exchequer. Socialists need to recognise these modifications, understand their significance and adapt policies and practices to them. Above all, the left needs to understand why the NHS that Bevan built can no longer stand unmodified. But first we must measure the extent of the modifications.

Politicians of the left encourage us to think of the NHS as an island of socialism in a capitalist sea. An imperfect beginning, it awaits the eruption that will extend it into a continent. The image is fanciful, and arguably wrong in one detail; the island is as much communist territory as socialist.

The distinction is important. The NHS is ostensibly available to all of us according to our need – a communist principle.[1] The socialist notion of 'from each according to ability, to each according to work' was avoided when the NHS was founded in 1948. Instead we have inherited an outwardly egalitarian health service in which access is divorced from contribution. Only education offers a similar gift of resources based on need. The remainder of the welfare state, and increasingly public facilities like housing and transport, provide minimum citizenship rights for those unable to do better for themselves. No one could claim that supplementary benefit is an egalitarian and redistributive form of welfare. Yet the premature baby needing special care gets it before paying a penny in direct or indirect taxation; its parents need not have paid VAT on a single packet of nappies before their baby is in its incubator. Nor is incubator space dependent upon the parents' future ability to pay. They need not be aristocrats, nor even labour aristocrats in a socialist economy. The baby qualifies for an incubator simply because it needs one.

This may not seem like a gift, but it is. Whilst it is true that the baby's parents will have paid tax on something, at some time, the NHS does not work on the basis of accumulated credit in the shape of past tax payments. It could not do so and remain egalitarian. Since we cannot predict what our need for medical services will be, and no one can predict the cost of it for us, we cannot store up money for future use. Taxation paid now is used now, providing today's services for today's ill, the majority of whom are elderly people no longer in the direct taxation income bracket. We all rely upon following generations to fund our health care when we need it, by their gifts of taxation. This is different from other benefits, like pensions, which are income-related and, in effect, accumulative. If the NHS worked on the same principle as state pensions, it would be more like an insurance-based system than one aiming at redistributing wealth to meet need. As we shall see, this gift relationship is the focus for the right's assault on the National Health Service.

Public Input

This common use of the common wealth is a just solution to problems of illness, but it has had consequences that many on the left prefer to ignore. For example, the absence of any notion of 'contribution' other than through taxation, expressed either as 'to each according to work' or as 'from each according to ability', has reduced public input to medical care to specific activities like blood transfusion, organ donorship, fund-raising for the local hospital's League of Friends, or membership of a special-interest group concerned with a particular problem.

These are significant forms of citizen involvement, but they are voluntary, not obligatory, and are subordinate to the main business of health care, which is conducted by professionals. As we shall see later, this has left the issue of participation open to the right's exploitation. Similarly, the meaning of the word 'need' has been assumed, not analysed, so that in practice it shades into consumerist 'wants' on the one hand, and into professional judgements of priority on the other. When commercial interests can influence or even define both public 'wants' and professional thinking, the concept of 'need' becomes compromised.

A second communist feature of the NHS stems from a principle stated clearly in the Beveridge Report in 1942:

> The primary interest of the Ministry of Health is not in the details of the national health service or in its financial arrangements. It is in finding a health service which will diminish disease by prevention and cure.[2]

Presumably a diminishing burden of disease would in turn require less of a health service, and so at least part of the state would begin to wither away. It is easy to be wise with hindsight, and easy now to parody expectations that seemed rational in the mid-1940s, but we now work with the health service that Beveridge and Bevan 'found', and to some extent with the assumptions about the effectiveness of 'prevention and cure' that they promoted. Disease is not diminishing, even though specific diseases are now preventable (diphtheria, polio), curable (pneumonia) or both (tuberculosis). Far from illness decreasing, the use of the NHS increases year by year, and the rising throughput of our hospitals has been projected by the Conservatives as a sign of government competence and care.[2]

All too many might conclude from this that Beveridge and Bevan were dangerous fellow-travellers, so impoverished is the political culture of Conservative Britain. Of course they were not, but they were expressions of two important and hopeful features of the left. First, the overlap in thinking about health between the subordinate, Marxist trend in British socialism and the dominant socialism of the Labour party, strongly influenced by Christian teaching. Secondly, the influence of these ideas across a broad political spectrum and a wide range of social classes is still so great that a radical right government has found it difficult to dislodge the NHS from public affection.[4]

Of course, the gift of free medical care seen by a communist as an emerging feature of a new society might be understood by a Christian as an expression of an eternal value, love, and the different philosophical approaches might have consequences for the future disposal of such gifts. Nevertheless, different understandings have converged on a single practice, the common use of the common wealth for the relief of illness. The possibility of finding common ground, both amongst socialists and in wider civil society, offers us scope for changing the way we live and making the communist principle of the health service sit easier in society. The endurance of a common practice in the gift of health care, despite the diverse origins of that practice, should be an antidote to the fashionably pessimistic perception of 'alliances' as being inherently unstable and therefore inferior to the pursuit of partisan interest. And the transformation of a utopian idea – a relationship free from money – into a real social institution that provides help, support, comfort and care twenty-four hours a day reveals the power latent within socialism.

A Free Service?

What has happened to the founding principles of the National Health Service? For increasing numbers of NHS users the service is not free at the time of need. The increase in prescription charges under Thatcher's government, from 20p per item in 1979 to 2.60p per item in April 1988, has created a two-tier service for almost all working adults. This conforms to the pattern of Conservative governments from 1951 onwards, which have tended to increase the proportion of NHS income derived from charges to patients, whilst Labour governments have reduced this proportion without ever abolishing it entirely.[5] On the top tier those fit enough to work must pay for prescribed medicines, unless they have one of a small number of exempt conditions like epilepsy or diabetes. On the bottom tier the poor, the elderly and children receive free medication.[6] Exemption from prescriptions is easier for some than others; those aged under sixteen and above retirement age being able to declare their exempt status, whilst those on low incomes or with 'exempt' conditions need to apply for exemption certificates. Inevitably, the process of application, linked to means-testing in some cases, leads to underclaiming.[7]

Spectacles are no longer available from the NHS, even for those on the lowest incomes, who must use vouchers to obtain services from the optical market-place. This change was introduced in 1983 to abolish the £17 million annual subsidy of NHS lenses by the DHSS, forcing the 3 million people opting for NHS glasses into the market-place. This reform took place in two stages, with NHS optical services initially restricted to children and those on social security before complete abolition of the subsidy occurred.[8]

Dentistry has an enlarging 'private' component, with a rising scale of fees paid by patients.[9] In early 1979 dental charges made up less than a fifth of the cost of the dental services administered by the Family Practitioner Committees. By the end of financial year 1984-85 charges contributed just over a quarter of the service budget, and by the end of the following financial year the proportion of the total cost of dental services approached one third.[10] Whilst the numbers of people exempt from dental charges because of low income rose from just over half a million in 1977 to just over 2 million in 1984, the total numbers exempt rose by only 400,000 because the age limit for exemption was dropped from twenty-one to sixteen.[11]

Residency qualifications applied in hospitals prevent citizens who are 'not normally resident' in the UK from free access to anything other than emergency care.[12] Victims of traffic accidents can be charged a fixed contribution towards the cost of out-patient care, and sums above this fixed charge can be passed on to a vehicle driver's insurance company, and can be extended to cover in-patient costs. In 1983 this charge contributed £10 million to the NHS budget, with significant variations between Health Authorities.[13] Even movement from one Health Authority to another can render a UK citizen liable to charges for at least one service – termination of pregnancy in areas where services are contracted out to charitable organisations.[14]

Family Practitioner Services

Charges to patients are much more significant within the Family Practitioner services (which administer general practitioners, dentists, opticians and pharmacists) than in the hospital sector. In 1984 the contribution of charges to service budgets was ten times greater for pharmaceuticals, and nearly forty times greater for dentistry and optical services, than it was for NHS hospitals.[15] This may explain why privatisation in hospitals takes the form of contracting-out an increasing range of sub-services within hospitals (from catering through diagnostic laboratory work to nursing), privatisation in the Family Practitioner Services has taken the form of increased patient charges, including vouchers for glasses and the abolition of free dental checks and eye tests announced in the 1987 White Paper on Primary Care, 'Promoting Better Health'.[16]

The temptation to extend charging from Family Practitioner services to the whole health service periodically overwhelms the Conservatives, but to date the flirtation has been brief. The Royal Commission on the NHS, which reported in 1979, calculated that a package of charges including hotel costs in hospital and fees for visiting GPs would yield about 8 per cent of total NHS expenditure, to be compared with the 2.7 per cent derived from charges in 1980.[17] In an authoritative review of alternative funding for the NHS, Butler and Vaile point out that whilst the savings achieved would be primarily from extra revenue, such a package of charges would produce some reduction in demand concentrated most heavily amongst those who could least afford to concede it, and cause financial problems for those who just fail to qualify for exemption on the grounds of low income.[18]

The Sigificance of Charges

So how much do charges really matter? There is a strong case against prescription charges on the grounds that they are unjust to those with long-term but non-exempt illnesses like asthma, eczema or high blood pressure, and uneconomic for the NHS compared with the possible savings from rationalised prescribing.[19] But are they a deterrent to treatment? The numbers of prescriptions issued and medicines prescribed has tended to increase, even during the recent periods when prescription charges have risen quickly.[20] It is tempting to argue from this that charges do not diminish overall demand for prescribable medicines.[21] However,the great majority of prescriptions dispensed in the UK are exempt charges, and the proportion dispensed free has risen significantly since 1979.[22] The limited effect of prescription charges on overall consumption of prescribed medicines does not mean that some have not found charges to be a deterrent, nor that charges as a whole are benign and without deterrent effect.[23]

For example, a Gallup poll conducted for the British Dental Association in 1983 showed that one adult in seven was putting off dental treatment because of costs.[24] The British Dental Association explained the sharp drop in fillings in 1985 as a public reaction to the 25 per cent increase in charges that had been introduced in April of that year, noting also that the slight increase in the number of people attending for dental checks indicated that treatment refusal occured once costs of treatment became clear. In 1981 the DHSS Dental Strategy Review Group warned that 'any charge to patients will deter some from seeking the treatment they need'.[25]

Charges have a complex effect on demand, dependent upon the problem and individual perceptions of it, the level of charge and the possibilities for exemption from it. Anecdotal evidence from pharmacists suggests that those deterred from cashing prescriptions are poor, with either long-term problems requiring regular prescriptions, or with episodic problems coinciding with a temporary cash crisis. The former group may be more important, in the long term, than the latter, since inconsistent use of medication for reasons of poverty may mean deteriorating lung function from under-treated asthma or higher risk of strokes, heart attacks or kidney failure from inadequately treated high blood pressure.

American experience of charges for 'health checks' suggests that fees reduce take-up of preventive services, and that take-up reduction may be greatest amongst those with low incomes, who also tend to be those with highest levels of preventable illness.[26] However,we cannot argue that zero fees produce maximum take-up of services. That is certainly not true of immunisation against whooping cough or measles, nor of cervical cytology screening, where uptake is well below 100 per cent despite free services. We can understand the complexity of 'need' if we examine these examples in more detail.

Take-up of a service may depend upon perceived value (low, in the case of whooping cough immunisation), costs in terms of time off work (and therefore lost income for some) and travel, and real or imagined discomforts and risks. These factors may vary according to the economic status of the individual. The manager may believe that 'time is money', but she will not lose income by going for a cervical smear, to which she can travel in a company car. The actual costs are so small, and the value so great that a fee for her cervical smear would not prevent her using the service. The packaging worker, on the other hand, may lose money by taking time off work and have to pay for transport to the service, which she may value less and fear more because her ideas about herself and her sexuality differ from those of the manager. For her, a charge would be an additional loss of income.

A Comprehensive Service?

The NHS in 1988 is much bigger institution than it was, and provides a much better service than it did in 1948, but it is still not comprehensive. There is no guarantee that specific services will be available in a given locality, and even if available, nothing to ensure their consistent accessibility.

At its foundation the health service inherited 1,143 voluntary (charitable) hospitals and 1,545 municipal hospitals, more than half of which had been built in the nineteenth century, and most of which were poorly equipped, even by the standards of post-war Britain.[27] The regional distribution of the nationalised voluntary and municipal hospitals reflected patterns of patronage and charity as well as municipal wealth and political control. London and Liverpool were well equipped with voluntary hospitals because of strong local traditions of philanthropy, whilst in London Labour-controlled councils had developed prestigious general hospitals around the city. Teaching hospitals were concentrated in inner-city areas that were soon to depopulate whilst long-stay psychiatry hospitals were on the outskirts of towns and cities in old Poor Law workhouses. There was no plan in the distribution of the hospitals of the new health service, and some of the best hospital facilities were available where they were least needed.[28] Early Ministry of Health policy concentrated on maintaining and improving the existing facilities rather than attempting any redistribution or rationalisation, and resources were allocated according to existing commitments, so perpetuating inequalities in provision. There was no 'grand strategy' for equalising provision before the mid-1970s, and even replacement of ageing buildings was delayed for over a decade, until the Hospital Plan of 1962.[29].

The NHS inherited the same variability in its general practitioner and dental services. Julian Tudor Hart's 'Inverse Care Law' was derived from his study of resource distribution within the NHS and states that the availabilty of good medical care varies inversely with the medical needs of the population served. A rider rarely quoted by academic users of the Inverse Care Law argues that this relationship is most strong where commercial forces operate.[30] Evidence supporting this law exists well into the 1980s, especially in primary care services in some inner-city areas – London and Glasgow in particular – but also in the regional distribution of hospital beds and general practitioners, in spending on community health services and even in health-related social services provision.[31] Dental services also follow the Inverse Care Law, with a disproportionate concentration of dentists in the South of England, lower patient-dentist ratios in urban than in rural areas, a social class gradient in use of services and similar maldistribution within both the community dental services (serving schoolchildren, mainly) and in wholly private dental care. This distribution pattern has changed for the better since the 1960s, but has yet to disappear.[32] A study of children's dental health published in 1975 found social class differences in parental knowledge about dental health, parental attitudes towards treatment, parental expectations about their children's future dental health, their children's use of dental services and the state of the children's teeth.[33]

People living within the territory of one health authority may not have access to the same quantity or quality of services as their neighbours in the adjacent health authority. Some variation in the provision of services is inevitable, since innovation cannot occur simultaneously everywhere, and some variation may be desirable, because experimentation with different approaches to care is essential. However, the variability of the NHS has, in the main, a less tolerable origin in the history and class geography of the nation. Use of health services is in large part determined by their availability, and not by the medical needs of local populations. In a situation in which services are provided on such a hit-and-miss basis, without prior measurement of needs, it is difficult to argue that the service is 'comprehensive', without making the word meaningless. What we can and must argue is that the NHS made more services available, without barrier, to more people than did the preceding systems in inter-war Britain, and that it remains a better structure for developing need-driven medical services than any insurance system or health maintainance organisation on offer from the right.

Nevertheless, we must acknowledge that half of the country's abortions, a quarter of hip replacement operations and most IVF treatment occur in the commercial sector, not in NHS hospitals.[34] Similarly, private provision of residential places for the elderly has increased from less than half that of the public sector in 1976 to nearly two thirds of public provision in 1984.[35]

Resource Redistribution

It is to the credit of its workers that in its first forty years the health service extended specialist care across the country, but no effort has been sufficient to correct the unequal distribution of resources inherited in 1948. The introduction of planned resource reallocation in the 1970s did something to equalise services, although budget restraints applied according to the formula of the 1976 Resource Allocation Working Party (RAWP) report have meant, in practice, more levelling downwards of Health Authority spending rather than the raising up of low spenders.[36] In some places reallocation policies have caused major problems. Regions like Oxford and the four Thames Regional Health Authorities with very small growth targets under the RAWP formula have found that their budgets have shrunk rather than grown once population migration and ageing and high local inflation in health care costs have had an impact.[37] Inequalities in provision may also have increased, particularly where community-oriented services have had to compete with specialist facilities.[38]

Despite attempts to equalise resources across the country, geography still matters. If you are born prematurely and need access to a ventilator in a Special Care Baby Unit, or have kidney failure needing dialysis, or have heart block correctable by pacemaker, try to be near one of the centres of excellence that can meet your need. If you have a hernia needing repair, or a hip worth replacing, choose to live in a Health Authority with short waiting lists. Whilst almost every citizen will get appropriate emergency medical care when it is needed, if necessary by transfer from one part of the country to another, routine services and even some life-saving facilities are not evenly and appropriately distributed.

The ensuing burden of tolerated or neglected disease experienced disproportionately by the working class undermines official claims of comprehensive provision.[39] In practice it has not proved possible to provide comprehensive services on the basis of each according to need, and socialists have been able to boast about our 'free' health service only by equating medical care with acute hospital medicine and general practice – an association encouraged by doctors of all political views. Services concerned with cure have dominated popular thinking to the detriment of those concerned with care. The measurement of needs and the matching of services to them has not been a priority either for the NHS or for the political movements that fashioned it. Judgements have been made on the simplest of criteria – the availabilty of hospitals to salvage (where possible) those already badly damaged, and the existence of a free diagnosis service in general practice. Needs are somehow supposed to get sorted out by this system, which functions on widespread public trust of professional decision-making.

Centrally Funded?

Exchequer funds supply most of the NHS's needs, but not all. Payments by users constitute just under 9 per cent of the total Family Practitioner Services budget, and just over

3 per cent of the total NHS budget.[40] To this income we must add the voluntary contributions made by citizens towards local health services. Without sponsored parachute jumps, fetes and direct appeals to the public there would be fewer body scanners, fewer day hospitals and fewer NHS hospice units.[41] Commercial videos played in overcrowded casualty departments augment cash-limited Health Authority budgets, and hard-pressed Health Authority managers divert time and energy into working out how hospital corridors can be converted into lucrative shopping malls.[42] Privately financed nursing homes siphon off the elderly infirm and some of those with long-term mental illness or handicap, using public money to support them.[43]

Private hospitals sell space and time in their underused operating suites to reduce NHS waiting lists, whilst agencies subsidised by charity perform half the country's abortions.[44] Nurses working for private agencies make good staff shortages throughout the NHS and at times can constitute the majority of staff on a ward or in a department. At different rates, and to different extents in different areas, the NHS is becoming part provider, part broker of medical care.

Implications

These changes in free use, service scope and funding have developed slowly since the introduction of prescription charges in 1951, gaining pace in the 1970s until they became a flood under Thatcher's administrations. But how much do they really matter? The statistics can be misleading. If the total contribution of charges to patients constitutes only 3 per cent of the NHS budget, it is hard to see charges as a major threat to the principle of free health care. That would be accurate, but for two trends in charging. First, charges are increasing faster than NHS spending, so that their small contribution to spending does not reveal their potential for growth as a source of revenue, just as the fact that until very recently commercial hospitals fielded only 5 per cent of the NHS bed complement fails to describe the commercial sector's dynamism and political significance.

At best the Conservative aim is to increase the contribution to health care derived directly from the public, whilst holding down spending on the NHS as low as possible, so repeating the approach taken in the 1950s. It is more likely that they are more ambitious than this, and are seeking to foster the view that users of the NHS are getting a service at too low a cost, thus making us all into claimants rathers than creditors despite our gift of tax for the common good. From this position flows the argument that prescription charges are just because they are less than the commercial cost of the medicines dispensed. As taxation falls and some people's personal disposable income rises, this argument begins to gain force. Those with the higher incomes are likely to have the lowest need for medical care and for prescribed medicines, and are well suited by the subsidised prescriptions that they occasionally need and can easily afford from their savings on taxation.

Secondly, existing charges to users are concentrated, firstly into the Family Practitioner Services, and then within them into dentistry and optical services. This concentration permits step-by-step change in the character of the service and experimentation with different approaches to funding. We have seen how optical services have been shifted out of the NHS almost entirely, and how they are likely to disappear altogether as part of free health care once the 1987 White Paper proposal to abolish free eye tests is implemented. The same process, involving gradual increases in charges and the elimination of free care, may be what is going on within dentistry. Rather than introduce a revolution in health care across all services, the Conservatives are feeling their way towards new systems of delivery and funding. Vouchers first appeared as a form of surrogate money to spend on social services, not in education but in the jewel in Labour's crown, the National Health Service. The resistance to them was fierce in Parliament but, apart from the optical bodies with direct interests, virtually non-existent outside.

Passivity

How is it possible for this government to proceed with staged retrogressive changes within the NHS without the development of a powerful response from the left and the labour movement? Although it is sometimes difficult to generate any active initiative from within the trade union movement and the parties of the left towards the problems of the NHS, that has not always been so, and the mass demonstrations of early 1988 suggest that it need not be so in the future. There is a hidden history of national and local campaigns against prescription charges and hospital closures, with the role of catalyst passing from the Socialist Medical Association in the 1950s to the far left in the 1970s, but with a few exceptions that history has been one of defensive efforts concentrated on the traditional core of the NHS, the hospital sector. No pickets have stood outside opticians, and consultations between the DHSS and the British Dental Association have escaped the lobbying that has become such a feature of Health Authority life.

The left has lost a major ideological battle by accepting in practice, if not in words, that some aspects of the NHS are more important than others. Our defeat began with the compromise over independent contractor status rather than salaried employment for general practitioners and dentists in 1948, establishing a forty-year experiment in contracting-out state-subsidised medical care that long preceeded the 'privatisation' of ancillary services in hospitals.[45] It has continued with the virtual elimination of optical services from the NHS and the shift of dentistry towards a half-way house between public and private care. For the health service the forward march of Labour halted, not in 1951 with the defeat of the Attlee government, but in 1949 with the introduction of enabling legislation to permit the levying of charges for treatment.

There has been a failure of vision that may yet cost us the whole institution of socialised medicine in Britain. The expectations of the left and the trade unions have always been less than those of the intellectual minority and the Marxist current within socialism, and the real achievement of the working class in imposing its desires on the post-war government was compromised by the conservatism of the desires themselves. Given the choice of an ideology that emphasised 'to each according to need', the corollary of 'from each according to ability' could have powered the extension of democracy into the control of the new society's medical services. There were precedents for this, both in the history of trade union influence over the 'panel' medicine that preceded the NHS and in the role played by trade unions in general social provision throughout Europe, but in the 1940s there were stronger countervailing pressures to accede to expertise and entrust professionals with the management of the new system.

The result within health care was institutionalised powerlessness. True, changes were made, and are continuing to be made, in the ways in which services are delivered, particularly in the care of ill children, in family planning and in maternity care, through the convergence of the interests of women and concerned professionals. That is a lesson that the orthodox political left still has to learn, but it does not negate the charge of institutionalised powerlessness. Access to decision making is shut off by a the very centralised apparatus that some socialists fought so hard to create, hoping that it would allow Labour governments to impose standards on local services in areas where Conservative majorities would dominate any form of elected management body and begrudge every penny spent. Combine that with the imbalance in knowledge and control between those who provide the services and those who use them, and we have a recipe for relative public passivity towards the problems of the NHS.

Passivity in that form does not mean that we are uninterested in health and illness as issues. On the contrary, the interest is enormous and is probably growing, fuelling a burgeoning 'health' industry that sells fitness and healthy diets, spurring the ambitious and entrepreneurial into becoming 'alternative practitioners' who can divine an individual's future, not from tea leaves or palm-reading, but from hair analysis or mineral assays of the blood. How many women's magazines lack a page or two on 'health'? Are television adverts for private health insurance talking to a uninterested market too passive to reach for a cheque book?

Consumerism has become the dominant expression of public awareness of and interest in health, partly because the restructuring of the economy has opened up services as commodity markets, and partly because there is no substantial cultural alternative on offer. We can recognise that when we see the radical intelligensia preaching to the working class about its collective experience of avoidable illness and premature death, and urging solutions that emphasise new roles for the experts with, in the most progressive versions, walk-on parts as 'participating patients' for the rest.

Within the health service the same passivity fuels the divide between professional organisations and trade unions, with the latter playing a restricted economic role and the former dominating debate on the ways in which services are delivered, workers are trained and technology is deployed. If opticians or retail pharmacists are members of trade unions, they join them as individuals driven by idiosyncratic ideological pressures rather than as an occupational group that identifies its interests in the collectivism of the labour movement. It is taken for granted that whole sections of the NHS workforce are, to all intents and purposes, outside the direct influence of trade unions and unworthy of more than fleeting interest. In such circumstances, is it surprising that the cottage-industry mentality of the independent contractor professions is so powerful? Even nurses, the largest professional group in the NHS and the occupational group pursued by the greatest number of organisations, have as their most disciplined, unified and ideologically coherent expression a professional organisation, the Royal College of Nursing, which is not a TUC-affiliated trade union.

Political Options

It is tempting to attribute the present political crisis around the health service, and the long-term failure of the left to retain control of its best invention, to malevolent Tory ideology (conveniently forgetting those changes introduced by Labour governments) and to imagine that all can be put right by a new kind of Labour government firmly committed to socialist policies. Nothing could be more unrealistic and inaccurate. Not only does this view overstate the power and significance for politics of Tory class hatred (and of ideology generally) but it also ignores the complexity of the problem that this and any successor government must face in dealing with the NHS. Socialist policies are of limited value without socialist practices, and socialist practice is unlikely to succeed if it cannot offer individuals better ways of living, and develop its own 'common-sense' justifications for leaving the old and adopting the new.

The reality is that the labour movement and the political parties of the left have tolerated a public-private mix in medical care virtually since the foundation of the health service. Socialists have assumed that the gift relationship must have limits, and never put the NHS high enough up the left's political agenda to have a sustained impact upon its development at any time since 1948. Whilst a new agenda for the left and a new cultural base for socialism may merge from the present political conflicts, rapid renewal seems unlikely. Given that background, and the changes that have already occurred in the health service, we must anticipate the continuation of some degree of public-private mix for the forseeable future, even if that is distressing to those of fundamentalist disposition. The desirable composition of that mix is open to debate, but in debating it we should be brave enough to ask a basic question. Is an institution designed for Britain in the 1930s suitable for Britain in the twenty-first century?

Notes and References

1 'In the higher phase of communist society, when the enslaving subordination of the individual to the division of labour, and with it the antithesis between mental and physical labour, has vanished; when labour is no longer merely a means of life but has become life's principal need; when the productive forces have also increased with the all-round development of the individual, and all the springs of co-operative wealth flow more abundantly – only then will it be possible completely to transcend the narrow outlook of bourgeois right, and only then will society be able to inscribe on its banners: From each according to his ability,to each according to his needs!' Karl Marx, *Critique of the Gotha Programme*, 1875. Henri Lefebvre makes a comment that is very relevant to this discussion of health care: 'A socialist society is still characterised by contracts and legal rights. According to Marx, it cannot transcend the "narrow horizon of bourgeois law", the odd mixture of formal equalities and actual inequalities this law regulates'. (*The Sociology of Marx*, Penguin, 1972, p.115)

2 Sir W. Beveridge, *Social Insurance and Allied Services*, HMSO, 1942.

3 Norman Fowler MP said to the 1986 Conservative Party Conference: 'When they [critics of the government] hear that in England last year we treated nearly 1 million more in-patient cases than in 1978, they dismiss that as statistics. When they hear that we treated 40,000 more day cases, they dismiss it as statistics. When they hear that we provided for over three and

one-quarter million more out-patient attendances, they dismiss it as statistics.' There is some justification for this dismissal. DHSS data on in-patient cases does not identify individual ill people, but admissions, and does not distinguish between admission for the same or different problems. It is possible that an ill person might be discharged too early because of pressure on beds and need to be readmitted soon afterwards because the original problem had not been resolved. These admissions would appear separately in DHSS counting, and might be seen as increased throughput, whilst in reality readmission reflects insufficient care initially. An analysis of in-patient records in Leicester Health Authority suggest that this is occuring on a significant scale. (James Jones, 'The Price of Early Discharge', *Health Service Journal*, 19 June 1986)

4 It is difficult to see this duality acknowledged. Commentators like David Stark-Murray, historian of the Socialist Medical Association, tend to offer a version of events that stresses orthodox Labour views of the evolution of the NHS. (David Stark-Murray, *Why a National Health Service?*, Pemberton Books, 1971) Frank Honigsbaum hints at the anti-Communism within the medical profession (Frank Honigsbaum, *The Division in British Medicine*, Kogan Page, 1979), but fuller and more balanced histories of the influence of the left and the Communist Party on the evolution of the NHS, and on medical thinking through the Sigerist Society, remain to be written.

5 See *Caring for Health: Dilemmas and Prospects*, Open University Press, 1985 and the updated graph from the same data on p.131 of *Facing the Figures*, Radical Statistics Health Group, 1987, for more details of levels of charges under Conservative and Labour administrations. The enabling legislation for charging patients was introduced in 1949 by Attlee's Labour government, which went on to introduce prescription charges in 1951, provoking the resignation of the architect of the NHS, Aneurin Bevan, and of a junior minister, Harold Wilson. Harold Wilson's government abolished prescription charges in 1964 but reintroduced them in 1966. For a fuller discussion of this, see Malcolm Wicks, *A Future For All: Do We Need a Welfare State?*, Penguin Books, 1987, pp.22-3.

6 Prescription charges increased 12 times between May 1979 and April 1988. Because of inflation the increase in real prescription costs is smaller than the rise in nominal costs, as shown in this table derived from table 5.14 of *Facing the Figures*, p.134. The 'nominal' column refers to the cash price of a prescription, the 'real' column to the price allowing for inflation.

Date	Prescription charge per item	
	Nominal	Real
May 1979	20p	20p
Dec 1980	£1.00	78p
Apr 1983	£1.40	91p
Apr 1985	£2.00	£1.18
Apr 1986	£2.20	£1.20
Apr 1987	£2.40	n.a.
Apr 1988	£2.60	n.a.

The difference between the real and nominal charges may be one factor which helps explain the lack of opposition the prescription charge increases.

7 See Alan Deacon and Jonathan Bradshaw, *Reserved for the Poor: The Means-Test in British Social Policy*, Basil Blackwell/Martin Robertson, 1983.

8 For a discussion of the background to this change, the financial and ideological motives of the government and the possible implications of the reform for both the public and the optical industries, see B. Griffith, S. Iliffe, G. Rayner, *Banking on Sickness: Commercial Medicine in Britain and the USA*, Lawrence & Wishart, 1987, pp.125-7.

9 Between May 1979 and April 1985 the maximum charge for routine dental

treatment increased from £5 to £17 plus 40 per cent of any additional cost over that figure. For more complicated treatments maximum charges increased from £30 to £115 (see Wicks op. cit.). Payments by patients for dental treatment increased from £38.3 million in 1976 to £217 million in 1986 (*New Society*, 23 October 1987).

10 See *Dental Health Services: An Opportunity for Change*, response of the British Dental Association to the government green paper on Primary Health Care, 1987.

11 See *Facing the Figures*, table 5.15, p.134.

12 These charges were introduced in October 1982 despite objections that they might harm race relations and cost more to administer than to collect. The expected yield from the first year was £6 million, but this was not achieved and the first six months of the scheme produced just over £374,000, with 69 of the NHS's 192 District Health Authorities collecting no money at all. Top of the league table at six months was Paddington DHA, which raised over £36,000, whilst bottom place amongst scorers went to Mid-Essex, with a levy of £4! (See *Defending the NHS*, Labour Research Department, 1984.)

13 Ibid. See p.16 for a further discussion of how this charge is operated.

14 Drawing boundaries around specific local health services has been done for years, particularly in the care of the elderly and in psychiatry, but such 'ring-fencing' became a sensitive political issue during the Conservative Party's Conference in 1982 when officers of Oxford Regional Health Authority published plans to meet their financial shortfall, including a provision to refuse treatment to people who were new arrivals to the Region. Whilst this resurrection of the Poor Law principle of returning beggars to their parish of origin has not become popular in the NHS, 'ring fencing' is still an option debated by hard-pressed Health Authorities ('Oxford and the Collapse of Planning', *Medicine in Society*, 1982, 9, 2, pp.17-28).

15 See *Facing the Figures*, table 5.12, p.132.

16 In other words, the government has pursued a traditional Conservative approach and to date broken no new ground in this aspect of its management of the NHS. 'Hotel' charges for hospital in-patients have long been an objective for the far right, but were repudiated by the Prime Minister herself in 1987, and the only major expansion of charges to hospital patients has come through the renewal of pay beds removed by the previous Labour governments. Family Practitioner Services, on the other hand, have a history of charges that make significant contributions to total budgets, and a tradition of Labour complicity in maintaining patient payment, whilst the Family Practitioner Services themselves have been contracted-out since 1948.

17 The Commission's calculations included prescription charges raised from 20p to 50p, a £20 board and lodging charge for hospital in-patients, a £5 fee for all visits to accident and emergency departments and £2 for a visit to a GP, but no change in dental or ophthalmic charges. (*Report of the Royal Commission on the National Health Service*, HMSO, 1979, pp.339-42)

18 J.R. Butler and M.S.B. Vaile, *Health and Health Services*, Routledge & Kegan Paul, 1984, p.67.

19 Substitution of generic medicines for branded drugs could save between £100 and £200 million according to J. Collier, A. McFarlane and J. Shulman, 'Prescription Charges', *Lancet*, 1986, i, p.967.

20 There was a fall in the number of items prescribed in 1979, but it began before prescription charges were increased from 20p to 45p in July 1979 and ended after charges rose to £1 per item in December 1980. Since 1980 there has been a rapid increase in the numbers of medicines and appliances prescribed, with only a brief downturn in 1984-85. (*Compendium of Health Statistics*, Office of Health Economics, 1987, figure 4.12)

21 See J. Curson and M. McKee, 'Charge into the Dark', *Health Services Journal*,

7 January 1988, p.19, who quote R.J. Lavers, *A Demand Model for Prescriptions*, Institute of Social and Economic Research, York University, 1977.

22 The proportion of prescriptions dispensed by FPC chemists without charge rose from 65 per cent in 1979 to 81 per cent between 1979 and 1986. Some of these prescriptions were free because those needing them had a prepayment certificate, allowing them to get medicines at 'bargain' prices by paying an advance lump sum charge to cover all prescriptions for six months or a year, but these were a small proportion of the total. Children under sixteen received an average of 4.3 prescriptions each in 1985 compared with 3.4 in 1979, whilst the retired received an average of 14.6 prescriptions each in 1985 compared with 12.5 in 1979. The government extended exemptions to the mothers of stillborn children in 1982. (*Compendium of Health Statistics*, Office of Health Economics, 1987, figures 4.13, 4.14, 4.12)

23 The effect of charges on prescription take-up has not been studied adequately, perhaps because it is difficult to distinguish between people who cannot afford to cash a prescription and those who do not wish to use a prescribed medication. One local study showed a 20 per cent discrepancy between prescriptions written by doctors and those prescribed by pharmacists, but noted that the missing prescriptions were most likely to be from semi- and unskilled workers, and to be for antibiotics and mood-altering drugs prescribed for problems seen by the doctors as relatively minor. See A. Rashid, 'Do Patients Cash Prescriptions?', *British Medical Journal*, 1982, 284, pp.24-6. This subject is reviewed in detail by Ann Cartwright, *Health Surveys*, King's Fund, 1983, with a plea for properly designed national surveys to clarify the situation.

24 18 per cent of women had put off treatment compared with 11 per cent of men, and 17 per cent of semi-skilled and unskilled workers had avoided treatment because costs compared with 11 per cent of managerial and professional workers. The high proportion of women deterred by charges was attributed to women putting housekeeping and family needs before spending on their own health care (*NHS Dental Treatment: What it Costs and How the Cost Has Risen*, British Dental Association, 1983).

25 *New Society*, 23 October 1987.

26 See Curson and McKee, op. cit.

27 See Brian Abel-Smith, *The National Health Service: The First 30 Years*; HMSO, 1978. Renewal of the nation's network of hospitals was one of the functions of the NHS Act of 1946, and nationalisation of all, including teaching hospitals, was accepted by the voluntary hospitals which needed financial support and had learned from the wartime Emergency Medical Service that state intervention did not necessarily undermine their autonomy. There was probably more resistance to this centralisation from Labour interests in local government, which wanted municipalisation not nationalisation and strongly influenced the then powerful Socialist Medical Association. We can only guess at the impact on service accessibility and availability if the NHS had been handed over to local government in 1948, instead of to the Ministry of Health. For a detailed history of this conflict, see Honigsbaum, op. cit., pp.290-1.

28 Aneurin Bevan's description of the inequalities in the new service is discussed in *Inequality Within Nations: Health and Inequality*, Open University, 1977.

29 This stagnant phase, from 1948 to 1962, coincided with Conservative governments anxious to hold down growth in public spending, and only ended with an upturn in the national economy. For a further discussion see Steve Iliffe, *The NHS – A Picture of Health?*, Lawrence & Wishart, 1983, Chapter 2. Policies towards hospital services, including the 1962 Hospital Plan, the centralising trend endorsed by the Bonham-Carter Report of 1969, and the reports on specialist facilities – the Platt Report on casualty services (1962)

and the Peel Report on maternity care (1970) – are discussed in detail in Robin Haynes, *The Geography of Health Services in Britain*, Croom Helm, 1987. Efforts to equalise services during the optimistic phase of hospital development in the 1960s did not necessarily achieve equality of access for the public. The Platt Report on casualty services reviewed the 789 casualty departments in hospitals in England and Wales and argued for a reduction in the number of such departments, with an increase in the size of those remaining. The report asserted that it was better for injured people to travel to a fully equipped centre than to use the nearby but poorly equipped local hospital as a casualty way-station for first aid treatment, but gave no evidence to support this argument. This logic, which has governed planning of accident and emergency services since 1962, conformed to orthodox thinking on hospital centralisation and the growth of District General Hospitals. The consequences have been to increase the costs of transport for injured people, to delay treatment through prolonged transport times (necessitating the development of rapid response emergency services that go to the injured) and to put considerable areas of Britain more than twenty miles from a casualty department, including most of the Scottish Highlands, large parts of Wales, most of North Devon and even parts of Norfolk and Eastern England. The number of casualty departments has fallen, from 265 major units in 1970 to less than 200 in 1982 (*The Hospitals and Health Services Yearbook 1984*, Institute of Health Service Administrators, 1984). This concentration of facilities has not reduced the number of people with minor injuries or minor medical problems from using casualty departments as primary care resources.

30 'In areas with most sickness and death, general practitioners have more work, larger lists, less hospital support, and inherit more clinically inefficient traditions of consultation than in the healthiest areas; and hospital doctors shoulder heavier case-loads with less staff and equipment, more obsolete buildings, and suffer recurrent crises in the availability of beds and replacement staff. These trends can be summed up as the inverse care law: that the availability of good medical care tends to vary inversely with the need of the population served.' Julian Tudor Hart, 'The Inverse Care Law', *Lancet*, 1971, 1, pp.405-12.

31 The relative poverty of health services in deprived inner-city areas is amply documented, as is the mismatch between the needs of populations with high proportions of solitary elderly people, single-parent families, the unemployed and those with chronic mental illness, and the high-tech specialist medicine offered by large hospitals. See, for example: Brian Jarman, *A Survey of Primary Care in London*, Royal College of General Practitioners, Occasional Paper 16, 1981; P.L. Knox, 'Medical Deprivation, Area Deprivation and Public Policy', *Social Science and Medicine*, 1979, 13, pp.111-21; *Primary Care in Inner London*, London Health Planning Consortium, 1979 (the Acheson Report); K.J. Bolden, *Inner Cities*, Royal College of General Practitioners, Occasional Paper 19, 1981. The lowest provision of general practitioners and hospital beds tends to occur in the poorest regions, according to B.E. Coates and E.M. Rawston, *Regional Variations in Britain: Selected Essays in Economic and Social Geography*, Batsford, 1971. Regional differences in spending on community health services are associated with the local class structure, with higher provision occurring in areas of higher social class. This relative underprovision of community services in predominantly working class areas also correlated with lower levels of hospital services. (J. Noyce *et al.*, 'Regional Variations in the Allocation of Financial Resources to the Community Health Services', *Lancet*, 1974, 1, pp.554-8). Tom Heller's study of East Anglian health services found the same picture, but made worse by the relatively low level of social services provision in areas underserviced by the NHS (Tom Heller, *Restructuring the Health Service*, Croom Helm, 1978). The

conclusion we can draw from these limited studies is that inadequacies in one area of the NHS are not balanced by extra provision in other areas, or in local authority care.

32 See Haynes, op.cit., pp.84-5.

33 J.E. Todd, *Children's Dental Health in England & Wales*, HMSO, 1975. Regions with the most tooth decay had the fewest dentists per head of population. A later study demonstrated that variations in use of dental services were not primarily due to differences in class attitude to treatment, but were related to the supply of dentists. In a town well supplied with dentists attendance rates were similar across social classes, but in a town poorly served there was a lower overall take-up of dental care that was most obvious in the children of semi- and unskilled working class families. Use of dental services was related to supply, but the strength of that relationship varied according to class. (D.M. O'Mullane and M.E. Robinson, 'The Distribution of Dentists and the Uptake of Dental Treatment by Schoolchildren in England', *Community Dentistry and Oral Epidemiology*, 1977, 5, pp.156-9). A similar pattern exists for adult dental health. The part of England and Wales with the highest number of residents per dentist in 1984 – 4,087 – was Yorkshire and Trent, whilst London and the South-East had the lowest figure, 2,677. The percentage of adults with no natural teeth was highest in Yorkshire and Humberside at 33 per cent compared with 17 per cent in London and 21 per cent in the South-East outside London. (*New Society*, 23 October 1987)

34 Private provision of abortions has increased since the 1967 Abortion Act. In 1968 35 per cent of all abortions were carried out in private clinics, but by 1971 the figure had risen to 43.4 per cent. Rudolph Klein points out that the 1967 Act made abortion legal and increased demand for the service, but the Ministry of Health set no guidelines for local health services to follow in providing clinic and operating-theatre time. The result was both the growth of private sector abortions and great regional variation in abortion services. In 1973 Newcastle region provided an NHS facility for nearly 90 per cent of women requesting abortion whilst Birmingham provided barely 20 per cent. Government reliance on 'clinical judgement' to decide on service provision permitted minimum spending, but this policy was only possible because the market was able to fill the gap. (Rudolph Klein, *The Politics of the National Health Service*, Longman, 1983, p.86)

35 Robert Maxwell quotes the following *Social Trends* data in 'Private Medicine and Public Policy', in *Health Care UK, 1987*, Policy Journals, p.83.

Residential accommodation for the elderly, UK, 1976-84, thousands of beds

	1976*	1981	1984
Private and voluntary	46.3	65.3	87.9
Local authority	105.6	121.7	120.9

* Figures refer to England and Wales only

36 The first attempt at resource reallocation was made in 1971, but was superseded by the report of the DHSS Resource Allocation Working Party (RAWP) in 1976. The RAWP report proposed the gradual standardisation of NHS provision across the country by a process of differential growth between Regional Health Authorities, based upon a formula that took into account the size, age structure and gender balance of local populations, their mortality rates (taken as the best available surrogate for illness patterns), movements of

people seeking treatment across NHS boundaries, teaching responsibilities and the value, age and state of NHS building stock. Similar formulae were derived for Scotland (SHARE), Wales (SCRAW) and Northern Ireland (PARR) and all have been the basis for resource redistribution between and to some extent within Regions, despite technical criticisms from many sources. For a detailed review see Haynes, op. cit., pp.36-52, and *RAW(P) Deals*, Radical Statistics Health Group, 1977.

37 See 'Oxford and the Collapse of Planning', loc. cit.

38 Tower Hamlets District, a socially deprived area within the Region losing most under the RAWP formula, cut beds used primarily for the social admission of people with poor home circumstances or insufficient social support rather than the new clinical block in the nearby teaching hospital. (J.S. Yudkin, 'Changing Patterns of Resource Allocation in a London Health District', *British Medical Journal*, 1978, 2, pp.1212-5)

39 The gap between the health experience of different social classes has widened further since the publication of the Black Report on Inequalities in Health in 1980. For one quarter of the population, the semi- and unskilled working class, rates of death in middle life amongst both men and women are nearly as bad as they were thirty or forty years ago, and for some diseases the problem is worse. The health of the professional, administrative and managerial classes continues to improve. Further evidence has emerged that the dominant cause of inequalities in rates of illness and premature death between classes is material deprivation, with lifestyle factors being a secondary contributor. (Peter Townsend, 'Poor Health' in *The Growing Divide: A Social Audit, 1979-87*, edited by Alan Walker and Carol Walker, Child Poverty Action Group poverty publication no. 72, 1987)

40 The income from charges as a proportion of total FPS spending is shown below:

1978-79	1983-84	1984-85
6.0	8.8	8.8

(Source: *Facing the Figures*, p.132)

Income from patient charges as a proportion of total NHS spending has increased from 2.25 per cent in 1979 to 3.2 per cent in 1987. (*Compendium of Health Statistics*, Office of Health Economics, 1987, table 2.7a)

41 Over 90 per cent of hospice care is provided by non-NHS services, which derive 40 per cent of their running costs from the NHS and the rest (plus capital) from charity, providing about 2,500 beds in 100 in-patient institutions. Located primarily in the more prosperous parts of the country, these non-profit private institutions run their own postgraduate training and have close links with the NHS, providing a model which the rest of the commercial medical sector seeks to emulate. (Maxwell, op. cit., p.80)

42 Mirra Holdings plc is reported to have identified 208 hospital sites in the UK and Eire on which it could build profitable shopping and sports centres. The company forecasts that twenty such centres will open by the end of 1988. The managing director, Robert Ainsworth, introduced the first commercial videos to NHS casualty departments at Whipps Cross Hospital, London (Peter Davies, 'What's Behind the Mirra Image?', *Health Services Journal*, 21 January 1988, pp.76-7).

43 The number of residents in private and voluntary nursing homes who claimed supplementary benefit rose from 7,000 in 1978 to 90,000 in 1986, increasing payments from £6 million to £460 million; Jonathan Bradshaw and Ian Gibbs, *Needs and Charges: A Study of Public Support for Private Residential Care,*

Avebury/Gower, 1988. The growth of private sector homes and hostels for mentally ill and mentally handicapped people has paralleled and sometimes exceeded growth of public sector provision, as the following table illustrates:

	thousands of places	
	1976*	1984
Mentally ill, private and voluntary	1.7	2.8
public sector	3.0	5.2
Mental handicap, private and voluntary	3.3	7.4
public sector	9.0	16.2

* England and Wales only
(Source: *Social Trends*)

44 South Lincolnshire Health Authority awarded a £100,000 contract for orthopaedic surgery to the commercial AMI Park Hospital in Nottingham in October 1987, using special money earmarked by the DHSS to reduce waiting lists. (*Health Services Journal*, 15 October 1987, p.1188) Oxfordshire Health Authority agreed in principle to a joint development of an extension to existing day-care surgery facilities with a commercial organisation specialising in private day-care surgery, Bioplan Holdings, having run out of the capacity to further reduce surgical waiting lists. (Barbara Miller, 'Private Profit Comes to the Aid of Public Service', *Health Services Journal*, 26 November 1987, pp.1372-3)

45 Dentistry is a good example of the distortion of care that can occur within a funding system that utilises market mechanisms. Dentists are paid for what they do, which tends to encourage intervention rather than a 'wait and see' approach, and they work as free-standing but potentially isolated businessmen rather than as NHS employees working within a professional career structure. Recent reviews of dental work have revealed a significant amount of deliberately unnecessary treatment, and a larger amount of unnecessary dental surgery performed because of obsolete treatment philosophies. This worries the government because of the costs (in 1984 one dentist made nearly £250,000 from the NHS) and should worry us because dental health is improving through fluoridation and reduced sugar consumption. (Jeremy Laurence, 'The Decay of the Dentist', *New Society*, 8 January 1988)

3 Twin Crises

There are two interconnected crises within the health service. One is a direct consequence of the economic recession and Conservative attempts to escape from it. The second is a long-term structural crisis of medicine itself, running over decades, and common to the advanced industrial economies of the capitalist world.

Welfare services throughout the capitalist economies have been reduced since the onset of international recession, following the oil price rises of 1973.[1] The specific features of this depression have had a direct impact on health services. Rapid growth of public debt encouraged governments to restrict government spending. Rates of growth of gross national product declined, with a 5 per cent fall in the combined GNP of the leading capitalist countries between 1973 and 1975, whilst world trade also declined and produced balance of payments deficits in vulnerable economies. Unemployment increased, reducing the tax base of public spending, boosting government expenditure on benefits and creating burdens of illness in the short, medium and long term.[2] Rising inflation increased health care costs, a trend made worse by the tendency of health service spending to have a higher 'internal' inflation rate than the rest of the economy.[3]

In Britain longer term economic trends combined with the recession of the 1970s to make cost-containment policies attractive to both Labour and Conservative governments. The orientation of British capital to overseas markets and investments, a costly obsession with international super-power status, the incomplete post-war renewal of industrial technology and plant (compared with that of Germany and Japan), a labour movement strengthened by wartime experience (again, unlike Germany and Japan) and a genuine labour shortage compared with the mass unemployment hidden within the more rural European societies, meant that Britain's economy failed to develop at the same rate as its competitors. This development, which occurred faster than in any previous period in the country's industrial history but still at a slower rate than in other economies, made Britain exceptionally vulnerable to the economic downturn of the 1970s. The recurrent political conflicts over funding the National Health Service that have plagued Thatcher's administrations stem from that vulnerability.[4]

The Second Crisis

The essence of the second crisis is this: whilst medicine has extended its influence enormously over our lives, it costs us all an increasing amount as well as costing more and more to get less and less individual benefit.

Now the overall per capita cost of medical care is rising, even though some medical practices (like heart surgery and renal dialysis) are now cheaper per person treated than they were a decade ago. The estimated NHS per capita spending on hospital services between 1975-76 and 1981-82 doubled for all age groups except for infants aged under four, for whom the increase was just below 100 per cent, and for those over 75, for whom spending more than doubled. The same doubling of spending for all age groups occurred in Family Practitioner Committee services (general practitioners, dentists, opticians and pharmacists).[6] This increase in per capita cost is occurring despite an increased throughput of hospital in-patients and out-patients, diminishing numbers of hospital beds, increasing deployment of specialised staff and investment of an increasing proportion of Gross National Product in the health service. The industrialisation of the NHS, with centralisation of facilities, better definition of staff functions, clearer demarcation of work tasks and speed-up of treatment processes has not reduced the unit costs for the most important unit of all, that of the individual needing the service.[7]

There are many reasons for the increase in health care

costs found throughout the capitalist economies. They are complex, interrelated and overlapping, and create difficulties for those planning or implementing policy.

Expansion of the services provided
The NHS at its foundation had no intensive care units, coronary care, massive laboratories, diagnostic imaging units, special care baby units and infertility and in vitro fertilisation services, or colposcopy (visualisation of the cervix) clinics and surgical lasers, all of which are highly capital intensive. Nor did it have psychosexual counselling, psychotherapy or other labour intensive services. It did have, and lose, lots of small hospitals and sanatoria, but they were primarily 'low-tech' institutions by comparison with their successors.

This expansion of services has in part grown out of technical advances – the X-ray camera combined with a computer to make a Computerised Tomography (CT) scanner – but it has also occurred because of shifts in the definition of illness and in the scope of medical intervention. The growth of consultations for psychological problems is an example of this, with consultation rates for neuroses, psychoses and alcoholism more than doubling between the National Morbidity Survey of 1955-56 and that of 1970-71. Consultations for minor problems increased faster than those for major psychiatric illnesses. The main response of the NHS to this constellation of problems has been to prescribe for them, so that use of mood-altering drugs has become widespread, with consequences for drug dependency, industrial and road accidents and hospital care of those accidentally or deliberately poisoned.[8]

An ageing society.
The increase in the proportions of the elderly and very elderly creates increased demand for services since these age-groups have higher levels of complex and interrelated illnesses than younger people. Whilst the significance of this factor is often overstated, since improved health through improved social circumstances means postponement of illness more than accretion of ill health, it remains a major contributor to increased costs. (The value

of these increased services to those receiving them may be arguable, but that is another issue and is dealt with later.)[9]

Higher pay for health workers
Whilst NHS workers' pay compares poorly with many jobs outside the health service, there has been an increase in both the incomes of NHS staff and the number of staff themselves. This applies not only to the professional categories but also to non-professional workers. For example, the catering, gardening, portering, cleaning and repair work was often done by able-bodied hospital inmates before final repeal of Poor Law provisions in 1936. The subsequent need to recruit and pay workers to do the jobs once done in return for accommodation by the very poor established a modern approach to organisation only a few years before the foundation of the NHS, and probably contributed to the financial problems of the hospital network that made its 'nationalisation' such a viable idea. This industrial development was continued during the labour shortage of the 1950s by overseas recruitment and expanded in the 'growth decade' from 1962 to the early 1970s.

Unionisation of the non-professional labour force in particular helped to increase incomes and with growing professional salaries pushed labour costs up to 70 per cent of the NHS budget. The growth of expenditure on wages and salaries has contributed to the above-average inflation of health service costs, mirroring the tendency of labour costs to exceed product costs in the post-war economy. The Royal Commission on the NHS estimated that 25 per cent of the growth in the real cost of the NHS since its foundation was due to this pay factor.[10]

New technology
The bulk of new services have depended upon new technologies supplied by commercial industries and applied, sometimes in a rapid and unplanned way, by enthusiastic professionals. These developments have done more than increase capital and running costs in every health authority. One reason why the costs of medical care are rising faster than the general rate of inflation is because the introduction of any new technique generates new, and

unplanned, activity that requires its own funding. A topical example are waiting lists for hip replacement, which have persisted and grown despite increases in resources available for orthopaedic surgery. This expansion made no difference to the hip-replacement waiting lists because the population needing such operations also grew, demand for surgery increased as the availability of the service became more widely known, and other problems competed for the time of surgeons and anaesthetists. Not only has the increase in the number of the very elderly increased the demand for hip-replacement surgery, since more people have arthritis for longer, but it has also increased the demand for for other kinds of orthopaedic operations because more elderly people – especially women – fracture limbs in relatively minor accidents.

Growth in professional activity
The increase in the number of doctors and dentists relative to the population has not only caused an increase in the labour costs of the NHS, but has also generated extra investigations and treatments. Tests and X-rays are used for more than the identification of pathological structures or processes. They can also be used to buy time, to amass data in the hopes of spotting a diagnosis within it, to be seen to be complete, to avoid litigation or just the prospect of being wrong, and to abolish the uncertainty of being without a diagnostic label. There are wide variations in the use of diagnostic tests betwen hospitals, apparently unrelated to variations in the mixture of problems dealt with, suggesting that there is no consensus amongst clinicians about clinical practice but reinforcing the idea that the primary determinant of service use is service availability.[11]

Market needs and effects
State agencies and contractors, including the NHS, play a supportive role to private industry, providing social capital for business in the form of improved health of the workforce and the consumer population together with a market for specialist goods, ranging from pharmaceutical products to the equipment needed for cook-chill catering. The state's health service also copes with the social consequences of

capitalism in crisis like increasing poverty, rising unemployment and persistent grassroots pressure for better services in a way that legitimises the state and the social order.
The very existence of the NHS shows that we have a 'caring
society' and obscures the uncaring economic mechanisms at
its centre.[12]

Accelerating Costs

This expansion in health service costs accelerated from
1950 to 1975, as is shown the table of averaged increases in
health care spending from ten advanced capitalist
economies:

Table 1

Changes in National Health Care Spending as a Percentage of GNP

	1950-55	1955-60	1960-65	1965-70	1970-75	1975-77
Average growth	0.3	0.65	0.64	0.94	1.36	0.15

Source: Robert Maxwell, *Health and Wealth: an International Study of Health
Care Spending*

Annual increases in expenditure on health services
consistently outstripped increases in national income, and
by the time the long post-war boom ended there was no sign
that the rise in health service costs would stop, let alone
decline. Since none of the factors driving expansion had
ceased functioning, there was no realistic expectation that
the apparently inexorable rise in costs could stop. The
response of governments was to reduce public expenditure
on health care, the Labour government led by James
Callaghan being one of the first to introduce cost-
containment measures.

The UK situation was different from the general. The rise
in the British health service spending rate was lower than
that of comparable European economies, annual health
service spending itself was lower than would be predicted
from Gross National Product and growth in spending had
started at a later date than in other societies. Compared
with most of western Europe, and certainly with the

highest spenders (Sweden in particular), the British government faced a small overspending problem, at least in the short term. Nevertheless the centralised system of control of the National Health Service allowed spending restrictions to be applied more rapidly than they could be in countries with insurance-based health services that give less scope for direct government intervention.[13]

After a brief interlude in the early 1980s during which NHS growth resumed, tight controls over spending have been continued as if the NHS had the same inherent problems as less well controlled and more market-oriented health services. Ironically, the ideas being considered by the government as possible solutions for an NHS spending 'crisis' that they have in part created derive from health services that are more prone to overspend than our centralised, public service.

Diminishing Returns

There is little evidence that this increasing expenditure of modern medical care is producing *comparable* improvements in general health. That does not mean that medicine does no good, let alone that it does little but harm, as Ivan Illich and the 'Disabling Professions' school argue, for everday experience shows that to be absurd.[14] The persistent high standing of the NHS in public thinking has something to do with the care and attention given to the ill, and the real improvements in the quality of life of so many individuals gained through the huge range of services – however patchy, incomplete and in need of improvement – that are available to those who need them.

Nevertheless, there is a problem of diminishing returns in medical care, and it has two aspects. It seems that we may need ever greater resources to obtain small improvements in the quality of life, and those resources are concentrated at the end of our lives in attempts at salvaging us from damage already done. In the 1970s massive increases in the numbers of NHS professionals and in the numbers of pathology requests, X-rays and physiotherapy treatments were accompanied by only modest increases in the total numbers of out-patients and in-patients treated, and a relative decrease in the number of new out-patients. The only significantly large growth in use occured with attendances at casualty departments.[15] At the moment no less than 70 per cent of all health service money is spent on the last six months of life. Less than 10 per cent is spent on health promotion, and equally small amounts go to the care of the chronically ill and the mentally handicapped. A recently published 33-year long study from Queen's University, Belfast, shows that people's average 'last stay' (before death) in hospital is increasing for women and has stayed unchanged for men since 1954.[16]

As new medical techniques are applied the gains made through treatment may become less than their economic, social and personal costs. Once a simple programme of immunisation could both eradicate a lethal infectious disease and make redundant all the costly facilities, staff and skills previously used up in feeble attempts at treatment. That is no longer possible.

Cervical Cancer Screening

One example of this is cytology screening for cervical cancer ('smear tests'), in which a 3.4 million increase in the number of tests done between 1979 and 1984 was accompanied by only a 9 per cent reduction in the death rate from the disease, a massive increase in the workload of screening clinics and laboratories, and an immeasurable amount of anxiety amongst healthy women at low risk of cervical cancer who waited, sometimes for months, to hear whether their result was negative or otherwise. The extra workload in analytic laboratories tested the quality of the service to breaking point, as happened in Liverpool when hundreds of smears had to be reviewed or repeated because of an inadequate initial assessment.

This level of pressure on the diagnostic service prompted knock-on demand for more laboratory facilities, which inadvertently increased demand as family planning nurses, clinic doctors and GPs who were attempting to limit smear tests amongst low-risk women because of bottlenecks in processing the smears found that the service had speeded up. For some of the educated, young, articulate and sexually active women whose anxiety about the rising numbers of their peer group developing cervical cell abnormalities or even overt cancer, the desire for an annual or even six-monthly smear test became a need. The smear tests done for them, sometimes in the NHS and sometimes privately, then took the form of tangible reassurances, performing the same function as consultations, examinations, investigations and prescriptions can do for 'well worried' people with other fears and problems.

Whilst reducing anxiety is a necessary function of the health service, it can also have a number of negative consequences. For the staff taking and reading the smear test, opportunities to do other work are lost, including seeking out those older and perhaps less well educated women with much higher risks of developing cervical cancer but lower motivation for seeking the test. For the women concerned this form of reassurance may mislead them about the accuracy of the test and the significance of cervical cell changes. Not only can this make it hard for women to understand why the health service may change its policy about the intervals between smears or about the time-lapse between the detection of abnormal cells and colposcopic treatment, but it may also have clinical implications.

Gynaecologists are quick to point out that apparently normal smear tests, or ones with only minor and potentially reversible cell changes, may not give a clear picture of underlying disease not identified by that particular test. Whether this detection failure is due to poor technique in performing the test or a feature of rapid cancerous change in cells in the cervix in some young women is unclear, but the outcome is the same. Diagnosis is delayed, sometimes beyond the point at which curative treatment can still be applied effectively, with the result that a young woman develops a cancer whose growth and spread can be slowed but not necessarily stopped.

Women learning this from the press, or from personal experience of a friend ill or dying from cervical cancer, are likely to want more resources devoted to training NHS staff to take better smears, more often, and they will be supported in this desire by clinicians dealing with this problem. They are not wrong to do so, but they form a powerful combined pressure group which excludes those women whose voice is not heard simply because they under-use the existing service, amongst whom there is a higher incidence of cancer of the cervix and a greater waste of life through late diagnosis of a treatable disease.

Earlier Diagnosis

The logic of seeking ever earlier diagnosis leads to the suggestion that colposcopy service itself should be extended out from specialist units into community-based sites, even though the cost implications for training and maintaining quality control of such a policy would make the current problems with smear tests look minor. This does not mean that smear tests are unimportant or that they should not be available to low-risk women, for the case for this preventive approach is good. The epidemic of sexually transmitted disease which began in the late 1960s, of which cervical cancer is one dimension (with human papilloma virus as the probable infective cause), will continue to claim thousands of women's lives well into the next century unless regular smear tests become a normal habit for young women now. Nevertheless the case for selective redirection of resources towards those of higher risk is better. If every woman over 35 who has not had a recent smear test has just one test soon, more women will live longer than if services continue their orientation towards demand.

This is a dangerous issue, since arguments for positive discrimination can draw the criticism of misogyny, especially when presented by a man. Yet a balance of distribution of resources must be found that reflects the interests of women as a whole, not just the young, and not just the most articulate in conjunction with the most powerful. We have grounds for being optimistic about this, because, of all the political trends on the left, the women's movement is most consistent in attention to health politics, most open to debate and diversity, and most commited to basing action on understanding not dogma. Neverthless, we should also note that the positive and powerful impact of the women's movement and feminism on health care has a consumerist dimension that may worsen rather than improve the health care available to some women.[5]

Heart Disease

Another example of this dilemma can be seen in the spectrum of medical responses to heart disease, from coronary-artery surgery to preventive strategies aimed at those as yet symptom-free. The beneficiaries of coronary-artery surgery are a small subgroup of a large population with heart disease, and the operations that prolong and improve their lives are no answer to the epidemic of ill health and premature death from coronary thrombosis in the larger population. Although coronary-artery bypass grafting (CABG) requires little equipment beyond that already available to cardiac surgeons, the more carefully the justifications for it are defined, the more limited it becomes as a practical response to the needs of ill or potentially ill people.

Whilst CABG has a place for those whose symptoms of angina are inadequately controlled by medical means, and also for those with signs associated with a high risk of a coronary within the next five to ten years, a development programme to increase facilities for CABG surgery along the lines proposed by the conference designed to produce a professional consensus on the issue in 1984 should be questioned. Is medical treatment being used sufficiently by doctors or by those with severe angina, or is surgery a way of short-cutting a laborious process of treatment that may, in the long run, give the same outcome to the individuals affected without the considerable risks of surgery itself? Will surgical treatment overshadow further development in medical treatment? What opportunities for developing preventive care on a mass scale will be missed if priority is given to the identification and surgical treatment of the minority with advanced disease?[17]

Even if we look at the medical contribution to prevention of heart disease, the probable yield on time, energy and money invested seems likely to be small. The risk factors most useful in predicting whether an individual will get heart disease are smoking and high blood pressure. Although there have been recent reports suggesting that medical intervention to stop smoking is more successful than initially thought, it is likely that high blood pressure is easier for health workers to identify, treat and monitor.[18]

Unfortunately medical control of high blood pressure, whilst possible and effective in preventing early death from strokes in those with very high blood pressure (at a price in terms of drug side-effects), is less succesful in reducing premature deaths from heart disease. A programme of prevention based on medical intervention against the two risk factors most closely connected with future heart disease would be compromised from the outset by the limited effectiveness of treatment for high blood pressure and the low success rate of medical help for those wanting to stop smoking.

The resource implications of such a programme, should it be pursued despite the low yield expected, are immense. An academic prediction of the resources needed for a one-to-one programme in the USA reveals the magnitude of the problem for health service planners. The study assume that there are about 7 million US citizens with arterial disease who are at high risk of a coronary, that 150,000 physicians (less than half the whole profession) are in a position to treat these high risk people, and that treatment is 100 per cent effective (unlike anything else in medicine) but must be continuous for one year. From these assumptions they estimate that there would be 84 million hours of consultations for coronary prevention alone, taking up something like 28 per cent of all physician time assuming a forty-hour working week and a fifty-week working year. This might seem feasible, even if the working hours are unrealistic, until the effect of new entrants to the at-risk population is considered. The authors of the study guess that 40 per cent of the US population aged over thirty has risk factors for heart disease – about 45 million people – and that caring for these people through blood pressure reduction, weight loss and encouragement to give up smoking as well as cholesterol control would use up 91 per cent of physician time every year.[19]

Delegation

There may be ways to avoid some of the workload implications of such an approach, by delegating screening and long-term care functions to nurse practitioners, who are cheaper to train and keep in post than doctors whilst producing the same or better results.[20] Some treatment, paticularly therapy to help smokers stop smoking, could be done in groups rather than individually, and treatment programmes could probably be streamlined.[21] Even so, the resources required will still be enormous. Since treatment of established disease is nowhere near 100 per cent effective without recurrence or relapse, and preventive care cannot stop all at-risk individuals from entering the high-risk group, the workload will not diminish as expected and premature deaths from coronaries will continue to occur. The case for getting more hands on deck to deal with this particular disease through conventional medical methods is not supported by our present knowledge or skills, particularly when the quality of medical care for relatively commonplace long-term conditions like asthma, diabetes, arthritis, thyroid disease and Parkinson's disease is less than optimal, when there are problems like pelvic inflammatory disease and low back pain that are widespread but poorly understood, and when special services like maternity care and care of the dying need considerable improvement.

This does not mean that medical intervention against heart disease is worthless. Coronary-artery bypass grafting has a place in the treatment of some types of advanced heart disease, and we need high-quality units that can provide accurate diagnosis and skilled surgery. There is a case for teaching cardiac resuscitation techniques to a wider range of health workers, and to the public. Progress in the development of drugs like aspirin which alter blood clotting may permit a preventive approach to heart attacks, or at least improve survival after a coronary. Rehabilitation after heart attacks is done inadequately in many hospitals, but can improve the quality of life enormously, and may even stave off later attacks.

At the preventive level every citizen should be offered a personal risk assessment, and help to reduce risk factors if they are high. To do this services must be both available and accessible; this has particular implications for people of different ethnic origins, occupations and educational backgrounds, and is also a medical justification for a universal service, freely available. Focussing attention on those with high risks where medical intervention (through blood-pressure control or reduction of cholesterol levels) may be helpful is a specific medical function which is likely to be both more thoroughly and systematically done by doctors or nurses than is an educational function designed to encourage much larger numbers of people to change aspects of their lifestyle.

Again, this does not mean that advice about healthy eating or exercise, or help with smoking or weight problems are topics that the NHS cannot touch. On the contrary, it is necessary to reinforce general messages about improving health with specific and personal ones that are of direct relevance to the individual. The point is that such reinforcement is necessary but in itself it is not sufficient to achieve the objective of a substantial reduction in heart disease. Other more powerful forces are needed to change the health of huge numbers of people. In a political climate in which state-run collective provision is diminishing and existing services are being overloaded we cannot afford the left-over aspirations of the 1970s, and must look for new resources to develop new approaches to health promotion and the prevention of disease.[22]

Health Promotion?

There will, nevertheless, continue to be pressure for expansion of services and staffing to accommodate extensive programmes of 'health promotion', with the prevention of heart disease the front runner. The government has signalled this expansion with its espousal of health promotion in the White Paper on Primary Care, and there is no shortage of professional self-interest already invested and ready to grow.[23] Of course, it is highly unlikely that any government will be able to pay for effective programmes against heart disease from public funds, in the forseeable future, for the reasons already given. Such preventive strategies will then face two options. Either to provide a service within existing resources, relying on the interest of the individual consumers to determine take-up of preventive care and the enthusiasm of health workers to shape provision of it, and so miss the opportunity to reach most of those most at need most of the time. Or to exploit external sources of extra money – basically private health insurance and individual incomes – to fund enlarged services which become increasingly like marketed commodities, and which exclude most of those at highest risk on cost grounds alone.

The existing models of medical care have a modest but significant contribution to make to preventing illness, but they can no longer serve as the template for all future growth in health care. This has been made clear through the work of the Swedish Future Studies Secretariat, which has examined the prospects for the Swedish welfare state as the twenty-first century approaches. It has found that:

> the number of people in Sweden over the age of 85 will grow by 70 per cent, from 100,000 to 170,000, by the turn of the century. Their current average annual in-patient stay in hospitals or nursing homes is two-and-a-half months, with lack of social support being a major factor in causing admission;

> life expectancy has almost ceased rising over the last twenty years, although expenditure on Swedish health services has sextupled;

> between one third and one half of all illness needing treatment is connected with the excessive use of alcohol;

> for every individual seeking health and medical care there is another person with similar problems who does not seek care;

> if the growth rate of the welfare sector in the 1970s were to continue until the turn of the century, running costs would quadruple, the welfare labour force would double to 1.5 million but the scope of activities would increase by only 50 per cent.

Britain is poorer than Sweden and has a cheaper health service, but the differences between the two nations do not erase the probable similarities in the underlying processes of social and health service development. The Futures Studies report has prompted wide debate in Europe, particularly amongst those on the left who look to Sweden as a model social democracy.[24]

Market Solutions

Only one solution permits the growth on a mass scale of low-yield orthodox medical approaches to current health problems, and that is the commercial strategy of 'creaming off' the healthiest sectors of the population and making them pay extra for medical care through private health insurance. Professional, managerial and white-collar workers have lower illness risks than skilled, semi-skilled and particularly unskilled workers, and it is possible to provide them with medical services profitably, at least within a range of relatively simple treatments for relatively common conditions. Those with adverse risks can either be charged more or refused insurance cover, as can those with existing long-term medical problems and those old enough to have rising risks of multiple ailments. This commercial approach has become viable because of the class variation in the overall improved health of the population. Whilst our health is improving overall, for the managerial and professional classes it is improving faster than for the working classes, and the poorest social classes are possibly as badly off in terms of health and illness as they were in the 1940s.[25]

This widening gap between the health experiences of different income groups does not mean, as some on the left almost seem to believe, that the rich and powerful never sicken and die, but it does mean that their chances of doing so within the normal working-life span are low. This risk is low enough to be spread across a population smaller than that covered by the NHS, so that the higher social classes can, through their collective better health, afford to create and fund a separate health service for their exclusive use. The insurance companies that finance and sometimes operate this service rely upon the larger and richer public sector health service to bear the costs of whatever illnesses and treatments are beyond the commercial sector's cash limits.

This is why the left is wrong to believe that commercial medicine cannot develop preventive services. It can, and is doing so, marketing attractive packages of tests and investigations that have all the trappings of modern scientific medicine but little of its real value. The wastefulness and irrelevance of commercial screening pro-grammes is immaterial once they become sought-after and therefore profitable commodities, since they pay for them-selves and do not have to compete for funding with other kinds of medical services aimed at other problems or age-groups. Not only does the busy young executive have no personal interest (yet) in provision for the demented, but also the commercial medical service which he patronises does not have to provide such a service for any of its customers.

The prospect, then, is that medical intervention against problems like heart disease is most likely to focus on those least likely to really need it, just as the middle classes get cervical smears whilst the working class get cervical can-cer.[26] The challenge for the left is to create the forms of health promotion that reach those at greatest risk as well as the greater number of those of lower risk. In political terms, this means expressing the ideas and attitudes that make different social classes function as one civil society, not different, co-existing but mutually hostile interest groups. This was achieved by the NHS at its outset, with the conver-gence of working-class, middle-class and professional inter-ests in a single state structure. It is being eroded now, with the growth of the affluent minority and the divergence of the health experiences of different classes.

'Getting Better, Feeling Worse?'

In Britain governments of both parties have had to address both the structural crisis of medicine and the economic crisis of capitalism simultaneously. Because the structural crisis is a feature of technological medicine, worsened by the operations of the modern market but not created by it, government responses to it have been similar, creating an element of bi-partisanship and of political convergence in government policy towards the NHS. The average observer then becomes confused. Why does one Labour government introduce prescription charges and another abolish them, only to re-introduce and further increase them, contrary to election promises? And why did a succession of Tory governments keep them constant until Margaret Thatch-er's administration promoted astonishing inflation, when both proclaimed the same objective of holding down costs?

One way to understand how the twin crises merge together is to look at this government's management of the NHS in more detail. The Conservatives have restricted public spending on the NHS to the point where services are now contracting. This is not just a simple attempt to roll back the welfare state because of its 'socialist' associations and its cost to the taxpayer, although certainly that is one motive. It is also an attempt to exploit one of the few areas of rapid development left open to capitalism in this country – the provision of services.

The epidemic of privately owned homes for the elderly infirm, funded by a mixture of DHSS benefit payments and bank loans, parallels the growth of private hospitals funded by insurance companies, medical co-operatives and US-based multinationals. The psychiatrists and psychiatric nurses baling out of the big mental illness hospitals to found profitable mini-institutions for ex-patients are literally cashing in on policies of 'care in the community'. Psychotherapists, alternative practitioners and assorted 'healers' are sweeping up the huge market for remedies, relief and reassurance that the NHS cannot satisfy. 'Health' has become a growth industry that needs an ailing public sector to thrive, and holding down NHS spending is a way of forcing the growth of private provision.

Productivity

The costs of the two most expensive areas of medicine – non-urgent surgery and long-term care of the elderly infirm – are slowly being transferred on a mass scale from the public to the private sector. Around them luxury private services – specialist medicine, allergy testing, 'natural' childbirth, psychiatry, screening clinics and the fringe therapies – are being developed for the affluent. The Conservatives are implementing the traditional socialist view that medical care can make a positive contribution to the national economy, rather than be a drain upon it, but they are doing so by promoting highly attractive but unrealistic individual solutions to social problems and concentrating on short-term advantage at the expense of longer-term costs.

That is not how Conservatives portray it, of course. They are able to proceed with the assault on the health service because they have been able to introduce a cluster of powerful ideas into common currency. Amongst these is the belief that the private enterprise is inherently productive whilst public enterprise is not. This view is supported by conventional government accounting methods which allocate all NHS spending to the 'expenditure' side of the account, but put commercial medical activity onto the 'income' page. This convention produces an absurdity. The in-patient unit caring for mentally handicapped people is non-productive when it is part of the public health service, but becomes a contributor to the Gross National Product once it is transformed into a privately owned, profit-making hostel, surviving on DHSS hand-outs and a big bank loan. If every ill person in the country were transferred overnight to a magically enlarged commercial sector, the national income would rise dramatically without a single change in medical activity, simply because commercial medicine costs its care in details that can be itemised on a bill. 'Productivity', in this sense, has no meaning for the NHS, which is concerned with different outcomes that are not necessarily financially quantifiable, and which may not be quantified even if quantifiable.

The health service becomes a 'burden' because it is supposedly unproductive, and that burden is felt in the reduction of personal income by taxation for the support of foolish people who continue to abuse their health despite sound advice. The sight of heavy smokers coughing, of crowded fast-food shops and of huge beer bellies propped against bars fuels the enthusiasm of the prudent, educationally privileged and physically fit for health insurance as a mechanism that would draw another line between themselves and their inferiors. The persistent high demand for medicines – particularly the largely useless ones like cough mixtures and vitamins, or the 'chemical crutch' types like tranquillisers and anti-depressants – reinforces the image of needy fecklessness that lies at the heart of Conservative visions of the working class. And, for the radical right at least, the irrationality of some current medical practice, and the huge variations between health authorities in workload, referral and care given are signs that the NHS is corrupted by professional self-interest, a doctors' gravy-train running at the taxpayers' expense but not necessarily for their benefit.

Infinite Demand

The huge numbers of consultations and prescriptions, of out-patient attendances and of people waiting for surgery, and the burgeoning of medical expertise into more and more areas of life, gives the impression that the slogan 'infinite demand, finite resources' might be true. It can feel true, in the chaos of the casualty department on Saturday night or in the seemingly endless queues for out-patient or surgery attention, but it is another absurdity. Demand cannot be infinite, since neither people nor ailments are infinite in number. Few like to seek help from the NHS, and many avoid it until they have no choice left. Most people with minor illnesses or mildly troublesome symptoms deal with their problem alone, or through the help of neighbours, family or friends. 'Infinite demand' is an arrogant exaggeration, the truth being that demand can be very great and can outrun supply. It does not always do so, as anyone working within the NHS on preventive care may have found, but it remains generally true that there exists undetected but treatable illness that is ignored despite its symptoms. If the word 'burden' has any value in health care, it is in describing this hidden disease and discomfort. Since the patterns of illness have shifted from infectious diseases towards 'degenerative' ones (like arthritis, heart disease and dementia), demand has changed its character, often faster than our centralised health service can change the orientation of its services. This uneven and delayed development means that mismatch of service to problem is possible even without government restriction of budgets.

'Finite resources' are the norm, not a notable exception, in any aspect of social activity, and there is nothing to be gained by applying such an obvious comment to the functioning of the health service. What might be said instead is that existing resources are misused and mismanaged, and that a fund of human labour is being wasted by a government that uses unemployment as an economic lever and a political weapon. Our resources are limited, but much less so than we think. This is unhappy thinking for the commercial sector, for which the 'finite resources' resources argument is a justification of their rationing of services by price, and allows them to 'cream off' the low-risk population and leave the high-risk population for an under-resourced NHS to manage. Or, as George Teeling-Smith, head of the pharmaceutical industry-funded Office of Health Economics, put it:

> Some people must walk while others can afford to travel by chauffeur-driven Rolls Royce. The existence of a majority of walkers should not be used as an argument against a minority of Rolls Royce passengers. Similarly, the miserable health status of some individuals is no argument against ... private medicine.[27]

If we do not appreciate the significance and substance of Conservative thinking and approach, the left may be marginalised and unable to influence future developments in the health service. The ideas that justify the erosion of the NHS are based on both experience and myth, and make some kind of sense of the contradictory character of current medical care. The left lacks the contrary views that make comparable sense, and can even be diverted into fruitless negations like 'finite need, infinite resources' for lack of more credible alternatives.[28] The strategy of commercialisation offers an apparent escape both from NHS underfunding and national recession, but it may have a long-term effect of increasing medical costs, so worsening the second, structural crisis, whilst it only solves the government's problems by transferring costs to commercial interests or directly to the public.[29] Nevertheless, it satisfies the narrow concerns of the affluent by restructuring health care in their interest, whilst contributing to the restructuring of the economy by providing a growth area for profitable investment. Any party seeking to replace the Conservatives in government will need a comparable strategy for health care that satisfies class interests as well as contributing to economic renewal.

Implications for the Left

If the logic of the situation favours commercialisation of medical care, with the development of a mediocre safety net service for the poor, why does Thatcher's government not intervene more aggressively than it does against the NHS, and shift the bulk of its work into the market-place? There are plenty on the far and not-so-far right who want to see more 'radicalism' in government policy towards health care, and whilst they have enjoyed some influence at times, it has tended to be at a distance, and with strategic rather than tactical thinking. Trips by Health Ministers to private clinics and hospitals, and the use of the commercial sector's services by the Prime Minister and, more recently, Health Minister Newton, have been propaganda for the entrepreneurs, but have never offset Conservative repetition that the NHS was safe, and expanding, in Thatcherite hands.[30]

There are electoral reasons for continued Conservative commitment to the NHS, even though this commitment appeared to decline following their 1987 General Election victory and the increasingly bitter campaign against inadequate funding in the winter of 1987-88, but there are also reasons within the structural crisis. The development of medicine has its own dynamic, which is in part dependent upon a partnership between professionalism and commercial interests. Professional workers in the NHS – in particular, doctors – determine costs of care by deciding on investigations and treatments for individual ill people. Despite their employee status British hospital doctors have a close relationship with the pharmaceutical industry, which is the main provider of postgraduate education, the predominate source of research funds and a major determinant of patterns of prescribing. This is the main link through which capital exerts control over medical care, shaping its direction and benefiting from its expansion. The industries which supply equipment – cardiac monitors, intensive care beds, incubators and so on – are a second route of influence. Such links are difficult for Conservatives to attack, since the NHS is the major market for these commercial interests and, in the case of the pharmaceutical industry, offers a pre-fixed rate of return on capital investment through a negotiated contract that permits prices of drugs to fluctuate to maintain approved levels of profitability.[31]

Commercial influence might not matter if medical science had reached its limits, but there is little sign that technological development in medicine is slowing down. Now in sight are:

> highly selective drugs that can reach specific targets within the body without affecting other tissues, or that can carry potent anti-cancer chemicals to malignant cells without harming normal tissue;[32]

> new developments in body imaging, giving more information about internal structures and processes than existing methods, more safely. Development of ultrasound techniques have extended this form of imaging internal organs both towards the very accurate scanning used to detect abnormalities of the fetal skeleton and towards the portable apparatus for bedside use. Magnetic resonance imaging (MRI) is being investigated as a complementary technique to computed tomography ('CT scanning'), with obvious advantages in fine detail imaging, particularly of the brain, heart and pelvic organs;[33]

> 'minimal intervention' surgery, in which the objective is to minimise the damage done to an individual needing some kind of operation by using rigid telescopes (laparoscopes) with small remote operating arms attached for work inside the abdomen, and flexible fibreoptic telescopes armed with biopsy tools or cutting lasers for work inside the intestines or lungs;[34]

> biological systems with the potential to identify and distinguish between chemicals in blood, or expired breath, or urine, making diagnosis easier, quicker and more accurate;[35]

> portable, desk-top equivalents of the larger-scale equipment currently used in centralised hospital laboratories for analysing blood specimens on a mass production basis;[36]

> information technologies dedicated to medicine, from simple computers capable of transmitting data from the largest Regional Health Authority to the smallest

clinic, to the possibility of complex programmes that make diagnoses as or more accurately than medical specialists.[37]

All of these will be extremely expensive, even when in mass production and wide-scale use. None of them may add as much as promised to medical care, except in special circumstances, but the commercial, professional and user pressure to deploy them widely will be intense. All are likely to distort health service planning by their work-generating effect on medical practice, and so could harm existing services.

The Disease Burden

The worst is yet to come. We are not running out of medical problems. Medicine is remarkable for the volume of unhelpful and ineffective (or even hazardous) work done by its practitioners whilst an enormous burden of unmet need remains untouched, even when the means and knowledge to deal with it exist. Old problems, like the medical consequences of high alcohol consumption, the effects of smoking (especially the tendency of women to smoke more heavily) and the impact of prolonged mass unemployment on health, seem to be increasing. Genuinely new problems are adding themselves to the list, with inevitable consequences for the organisation of medical care. The latest of the waves of ill health are the sexually transmitted diseases, of which cervical cancer affecting young women and AIDS, affecting almost anybody, are the most frightening examples.

We have seen how a screening programme for young women at lower risk of developing cervical cancer is important, because if it is not operating soon the cohort of women who became sexually active in the late 1960s and early 1970s will enter the high-risk age range for cervical cancer without having aquired the habit of having regular smear tests, and without having a mechanism to offer them suitable, regular reminders. An increase in the numbers of women dying from this avoidable disease could occur around the turn of the century. If sexual behaviour does not change to reduce risks of transmission of the probable causal agent of cervical cancer, human papilloma virus, that increased death rate will be continued by a further cohort of victims.

Epidemic AIDS

We cannot yet predict the effects of the AIDS virus or the extent of its spread, but we know that a few hundred seriously ill sufferers can overload a Health Authority that seeks to provide them with care that is sometimes all too basic. The key variables that predict the likely spread of HIV (the AIDS virus) remain unknown quantities, and it is possible that it may take between thirty and fifty years to learn about them.[38] We do not know the numbers of people carrying the virus, and for technical reasons would not find out even by testing the whole population, even assuming that such an approach would be politically tolerable.[39] The degree and duration of infectivity of those carrying the AIDS virus is not yet known; nor is the interaction between the infected group of the population and those not (yet) infected. The precise levels of risk of catching HIV through sexual activity and the real value of efforts to change sexual behaviour, particularly amongst heterosexuals, remain uncertain.

Estimates of the scope of the coming AIDS epidemic are, therefore, little more than guesses which are sometimes ideologically motivated. The Christian Medical Fellowship's book *The 20th Century Plague* suggests that up to 3 million UK citizens could carry HIV by 1991, rising to 12 million by 1994, most of whom would constitute a symptom-free 'time bomb' ready to explode early in the twenty-first century. A less doom-laden scenario, which assumes that the virus does not spread significantly beyond the homosexual population predicts that the epidemic's peak will be in 1998, when 48,000 will be dying from AIDS and another 60,000 will be suffering less severe forms of the illness. Thereafter the annual death rate would fall towards 7,000 or 8,000. This estimate could hardly be called optimistic, but it may underestimate the likely spread amongst heterosexuals, for the virus might spread rapidly amongst those who have large numbers of sexual partners. It would only need a proportion of these individuals to become symptom-free carriers for a long period of time for the virus to disseminate, slowly, amongst sections of the population with lower rates of change of sexual partner.[40]

Political Dilemmas

Now we can see the Conservatives' dilemma. New health risks are appearing, as if we did not have enough already. The existing services grow with a mind of their own as capital encourages professional enthusiasm, and outrun the (public) money supply despite the inherent power of the NHS to constrain over-exuberant growth. The benefits of medicine, in economic terms, do not add up to as much as the costs. Since they cannot attack capital easily, the Conservatives have to rely on market mechanisms to regulate medical expenditure. Operations will be done, people will feel well or ill, according to the profitability of this treatment or that. Commercialisation of medicine is, for a political tradition with no new ideas, the only conceivable source of new resources and therefore the only logical step. Fortunately, we can do better.

Notes and References

1 'Cost containment' has become a health policy theme for all west European governments, with a variety of methods used, some of which have been described in part 1. Brian Abel-Smith analyses these methods and policies, and their implications, in *Cost Containment in Health Care: A Study of 12 European Countries 1977-83*, Occasional Papers on Social Administration No. 73, Bedford Square Press/NCVO, 1984.

2 The evidence linking unemployment with ill-health is summarised in Riochard Smith, *Unemployment and Health: A Disaster and a Challenge*, OUP, 1987.

3 For a fuller discussion of the political economy of health in the context of the economic problems of capitalism, see Vicente Navarro, 'The Crisis of the International Capitalist Order and its Implications for the Welfare State' in *Issues in the Political Economy of Health Care*, editor J.B.McKinlay, Tavistock, 1984.

4 The peculiarities of the UK economy in the recession are analysed at length in David Currie, 'World Capitalism in Recession', in *The Politics of Thatcherism*, editors Stuart Hall and Martin Jacques, Lawrence & Wishart, 1983. He includes a significant and prophetic comment on the Alternative Economic Strategy of the left: 'By reversing cuts in the public sector, and indeed aiming for further expansion, the AES involves a significant expansion of public sector employment, so that unemployment can be cut to acceptable levels ... But this is not without its attendant dangers. For it implies that the main thrust of

expansion will be in the public sector, not in a greatly increased supply of industrial goods. And this means that any short-term rise in take-home pay will have to be restricted, with the fruits of the expansion being enjoyed in the form of a rise in the social provision of services (i.e., the social wage). This need not be unappealing, particularly since the left should be able to devise imaginative new forms of social provision ... to replace the atomistic structure of many parts of our lives under contemporary capitalism. But this requirement needs to be considered carefully and absorbed into our political campaigning if false expectations are not to be aroused.' (p.103) Imaginative new forms of social provision of left inspiration are short on the ground, careful consideration has been given low priority and the Alternative Economic Strategy is now off the left's agenda.

5 This is attributed to the failure of the screening service to reach those women at highest risk – working-class women over forty with large families, as well as younger women who have more sexual partners – and the blame is laid at the door of general practitioners for failing to reach the at-risk groups. 'There is a minority of women over 40 who are very resistant to having a smear and it is in this age group that 90 per cent of deaths occur. GPs could pounce on them when they come to the surgery,' says Dr Robert Yule, consultant cytopathologist at the biggest smear test laboratory in Britain, in Manchester's Christie Hospital (*Pulse*, 9 August 1986). A more analytic view is taken by Jeremy Laurance ('The Cervical Cancer Scandal', *New Society*, 16 October 1987), who points out that the age distribution of the disease is shifting towards younger women and the incidence amongst them of cervical cancer is rising, that errors in taking, interpreting and following up the tests done can be astonishingly high, and the bottlenecks at treatment stage compromise the whole screening programme by delaying necessary therapy. He says that 'the failure of the cervical cancer screening programme mirrors the "failure" of the NHS. Instead of reducing disease, and hence demand, more and more money is being spent with little apparent beneficial effect. Other countries appear to do things better with the same money. In the light of this it would be folly to expand the service until we have improved the one we have so that it is working as it should.'

6 See Figures 2.12 and 2.13, *Compendium of Health Statistics*, Office of Health Economics, 1987. The total cost of the NHS rose by £16 billion between 1949 and 1983, at then current prices, and doubled in cost when spending is expressed in terms of 1949 constant prices. The percentage of GNP spent on the NHS rose from 4 in 1949 to over 6 in 1983 (ibid., Figure 2.9). The proportion of this expenditure allocated to hospital services rose from 53 to 61 per cent over the same timescale, despite official commitment to community-based care (ibid., Figure 3.1).

7 The number of new hospital out-patient cases per 1,000 UK residents rose from 271 in 1954 to 376 in 1981, whilst the numbers of discharges and deaths per available bed rose from 7.6 to 15.9 over the same time period (ibid., Tables 3.25 and 3.38). The average number of hospital beds available each day fell by 11 per cent between 1974 and 1981, and the average length of in-patient stay fell by 21 per cent over the same period (ibid., Tables 3.16 and 3.29). The number of hospital medical staff grew by 25 per cent, whilst the numbers of nurses and midwives rose from just under 410,000 to just over 520,000 (ibid., Table 3.10).

8 Whether this trend constituted the exposure of a hidden burden of ill health needing attention or the 'medicalisation' of the usual difficulties and unhappiness of everyday life is discussed in Chapter 8 of Agnes Miles, *The Mentally Ill in Contemporary Society*, Basil Blackwell, 1987. The nature of the process may be less important than its outcomes, which include a rising consumption of mood-altering drugs with consequent problems of drug

dependence, and reinforcement of the idea of indefinite progress, with problems becoming increasingly amenable to solution through expert intervention. This phase of rationalist thinking may be ending, since prescribing of mood altering drugs had decreased since the mid-1970s, as this table shows:

Prescription issued	percentage change, 1975 -1982
Sleeping tablets	– 0
Anti-depressants	– 8
Tranquillisers	–13

(Source: *Compendium of Health Statistics*)

However, the reduction in prescribing may mask a transfer of responsibilities and functions to counsellors, social workers, clinical psychologists and psychotherapists, and a move by sections of the public disillusioned by modern pharmaceutical solutions to alternative practitioners.

9 The projected increase in the numbers of people over 75 is expected to double the workload of general practitioners by 1990. It is the over-75s who need and use medical services at a high level, whilst those under 75 but past retirement age do not have a greatly different pattern of illness than younger adults. Whilst the growth in numbers is greatest amongst the over-75s, the greatest percentage growth will be amongst the over-85s, who will form an enlarging proportion of the population until after 2011. The 'dependency ratio' (the number of over 65s per 100 aged 16-64) is high in Britain at around 23, with implications for living standards of all. (M.K. Thomson, *The Care of the Elderly in General Practice*, Churchill Livingstone, 1984, pp.3-9)

10 Pay policy in the NHS is a complicated topic, and not just because of the differentials between different grades of workers. The low costs of the NHS compared with European health services derive in part from the ability of government to hold down NHS staff incomes. During the 1950s the real incomes of hospital administrators and GPs fell by about 20 per cent, just as the real average income of the working population was rising by the same proportion. (See Rudolph Klein, *The Politics of the National Health Service*, Longman, 1983, p.56) The subsequent successful efforts by professional organisations to increase their members' incomes were followed by the growth of trades unionism throughout the NHS in the 1970s, summarised in Mick Carpenter, 'The labour movement in the National Health Service', in *Industrial Relations and Health Services*, editors Amarjit Singh Sethi and Stuart Dimmock, Croom Helm, 1982. Since labour costs have increased faster than the costs of goods for most of the lifetime of the NHS, the health service has tended to become more costly (compared with the general trend in prices) over a long period of time. This has contributed to the particularly high level of inflation within the NHS, and may have constituted 25 per cent of the real increase in health service expenditure between 1950 and the late 1970s. (See J.R. Butler and M.S.B. Vaile, *Health and Health Services*, Routledge & Kegan Paul, 1984, p.54.)

11 Bryan Jennett discusses inappropriate investigation in detail in Chapter 3 of *High Technology Medicine*.

12 These roles enhance the expansionary trends inherent within the welfare state but create their own economic crisis as the rising taxation necessary to permit public sector growth challenges both personal incomes and industrial profits. This Marxist view, derived from an analysis of post-war advanced capitalist economies, presents welfare states as balancing mechanisms that correct for the inherent instability of the market economy, but this does not

explain the apparent relative autonomy of interest groups within the welfare apparatus itself. 'Empire building' by those providing the service, supported (up to a point) by those using it, can occur through 'political advertising' in the form of party policy, government statements and the reports of official commissions and public enquiries. One example of this process is the remarkable speed with which maternity care was centralised in hospitals, with government policy and opinion following behind professional judgement that was itself only partly based on scientific thinking. See Butler and Vaile, op. cit., pp.60-1 for a discussion of Marxist and 'political advertising' theories, and Alison Macfarlane and Rona Campbell, *Where to be Born? The Debate and the Evidence*, National Perinatal Epidemiology Unit, 1987.

13 These are average growth figures for the ten-country study reported in Robert Maxwell's *Health and Wealth: An International Study of Health Care Spending*, Lexington Books, 1981. The same trends appear in the NHS, but are much less apparent than they are in, say, the Swedish or US health care systems. Health service expenditure in Britain started to increase later than other countries, grew at a slower rate, and began to decline once remedial policies were introduced by a Labour government in the mid-1970s, as the following table derived from Table 5.1 of Maxwell's study shows.

Growth in NHS spending as a percentage of GNP

1950-55	1955-60	1960-65	1965-70	1970-75	1975-77
-0.5	+0.4	+0.1	+0.4	+1.2	-0.3

However, the early restraint on NHS spending was short-lived, and the proportion of GNP going to the health service began to rise again after 1979.

NHS expenditure as a percentage of GNP

1977	1978	1979	1980	1981	1982
5.2	5.2	5.2	5.8	6.1	6.0

(Source: *Cost Containment in Health Care: A Study of 12 European Countries*, Brian Abel-Smith, Bedford Square Press/NCVO, 1984. The figures apply to the NHS in England only.)

This later increase in expenditure put the UK (along with France) ahead of other EEC countries in the rate of growth of health service spending, despite our initial slow start.

Average annual growth rates in GNP percentage
devoted to health care

	1966-75	1977-82
Denmark	6.7	nil (1979-82 data)
West Germany	7.4	1.2
France	3.5	3.8
Ireland	9.3	5.7
Italy	6.9	2.3
Luxembourg	7.4	4.6
Netherlands	6.1 (1970-76 data)	2.6
UK	2.8	3.1

(Source: Ibid. Table 1.1, p.33.)

Interpreting these differences is difficult. The differences in the definition of health care in different countries can be so great that international comparisons may not be comparing like with like. Even when great efforts have been made to compensate for this, as in Robert Maxwell's study, the results may ambiguous. Does Britain's slow start to growth and low baseline of investment, attributable to centralised control and funding, permit sustained NHS growth (in terms of GNP percentage used) when other countries with cruder control mechanisms over semi-private systems are reducing expenditure dramatically? Or does the continued increase in GNP spent on the NHS imply that the control that restrained spending in the past has failed?

14 Ivan Illich takes Bernard Shaw's aphorism that the medical profession is a conspiracy against the laity to its extreme, and argues forcefully that it is *nothing but* a conspiracy to which we are all victims. This reduction of all powers and forces to one, an overwhelmingly dominant group that controls the minds and lives of a huge mass of subordinate people seems to have great appeal, both on the left and the right. Perhaps it reflects the wishful thinking of the authoritarian mind, but it certainly is not an accurate description of modern social life, however true some of its details may be. The observable fact that medicine may act as a conspiracy against the laity does not mean that it always does so, or that it can do no other. See *Medical Nemesis: The Expropriation of Health*, Ivan Illich, Calder & Boyars, 1975, and *Disabling Professions*, Ivan Illich (editor), Marion Boyars, 1977. A detailed rebuttal of the Illich approach can be found in David Horrobin, *Medical Hubris: A Reply to Ivan Illich*, Churchill Livingstone, 1977.

15 See Stuart Haywood and Andy Alaszewski, *Crisis in the NHS*, Croom Helm, 1980, p.104 and Figure 5.2. This diminished 'productivity' has encouraged the present government to squeeze more work out of NHS staff and concentrate on crude throughput figures as if they were some rational measure of the value of medical care. By an irony of history simple socialist planning indicators have been imported to the NHS from the early Soviet five-year plans by a government keen to roll back the frontiers of socialism. Just as Soviet production of, say, nails was once measured in terms of 'nail-tons', allowing a factory to meet its quota by producing one massive nail, so Conservative Health Ministers urge us to count the number of in-patient admissions (not even the number of people!) without considering the quality of care received or the outcome for their health.

16 See Astrid Heiberg, 'The Doctor in the Twenty-first Century', *British Medical Journal*, 1987, 295, pp.1602-3 and Robert Stout and Vivienne Crawford, *Lancet*, 2 Febuary 1988.

17 CABG is examined at length in Jennett, op. cit. Jennett describes the different rates of development of CABG techniques in Britain and the USA, noting that slower take-up of this approach in Britain was almost certainly due to the more limited resources available to the NHS. His cost-benefit analysis of CABG suggests that for highly selected individuals with severe disease the technique gives greater value for money than, say, kidney dialysis. (See pp.104-11 and 164-6.)

18 Chris Donovan's leading article 'Prevention in Practice: A New Initiative', *British Medical Journal*, 1988, 296, p.312) reviews the medical literature and gives success rates of medical advice designed to help to smokers to stop smoking, ranging from 9 to 27 per cent. Success is defined as one year's cessation of smoking; longer-term success rates, if any, are as yet unknown.

19 'Epidemiology and Health Policy: Coronary Heart Disease' by Leonard Syme and Jack Guralnik, in *Epidemiology and Health Policy*, editors Sol Levine and Abraham Lilienfeld, Tavistock 1987. They point out that most of the input in policy formation for strategies to reduce heart disease comes from physicians who may be both unfamiliar and uncomfortable with known coronary risk

factors like stress, physical activity and obesity, and who are likely to emphasise approaches over which doctors have control rather than social policy changes beyond professional control.

This theme is explored in greater depth by Wendy Farrant and Jill Russell in *The Politics of Health Information*, Bedford Way Papers No. 28, 1986. They review the scientific evidence about the causes of heart disease, and the scope for prevention, and highlight ways in which the current scientific consensus illustrates the ways in which knowledge is socially constructed, with governmental, commercial and professional interests moulding a perception of the heart disease problem in terms that are individualistic and behaviour-oriented. This denial of social factors in disease creation makes orthodox thinking about heart disease as much an ideology that reinforces current values and attitudes as a scientific theory that clarifies the problem, they argue, and by encouraging a victim-blaming, top-down, dogmatic and prescriptive approach undermines the very effectiveness of the health education which it promotes.

They call for 'a style of health education that is more intellectually honest in its reflection of epidemiological evidence, and more sensitive, appropriate and empowering to the lives of the individuals it addresses'. (p.61) Interestingly, there are signs of a shift in orthodox medical thinking about risk factors for heart disease. A *British Medical Journal* leader, 'Refining Thinking on Type A Behaviour and Coronary Heart Disease' by psychiatrist Tom Sensky (1987, 295, pp.69-70) discussed the research findings linking heart attacks to behaviour and personality, and urged further investigation in the form of intervention studies designed to see if illness through heart disease can be reduced by psychological methods.

20 A review of nurse practitioner experiments is given by Andrew Long and Geoffrey Mercer in Chapter 11 of *Health Manpower: Planning, Production and Management*, Croom Helm, 1987. They discuss Barbara Stilwell's Birmingham Project and Barbara Burke-Master's East London Project, comment on the Cumberledge Report (*Neighbourhood Nursing – A Focus for Care*) and quote extensively from Julian Tudor Hart, 'Practice Nurses: An Underused Resource', *British Medical Journal*, 1985, 290, pp.1162-3.

21 Bobbie Jacobson discusses the advantages of self-help groups in *Beating the Ladykillers: Women and Smoking*, Pluto Press, 1986. The 'smokers awareness quiz', 'personal risk profile' and 'confidence test' she includes in Chapter 11 could be used in group settings as well as individually. Obesity is also amenable to change through group approaches, where mutual support, group pressure and competition can operate in a positive way. See J.S. Garrow, *Treat Obesity Seriously*, Churchill Livingstone, 1981.

22 The Coronary Prevention Group argues that strategies aimed at whole populations and at high-risk individuals or families are complementary, not alternative approaches, and recommends a number of 'good practices' within the NHS that it believes would facilitate both strategies. Unfortunately its recommendations are a shopping list of desireable services whose financial costs and opportunity costs are not given. See 'Risk Assessment: Its Role in the Prevention of Coronary Heart Disease: Recommendations of the Scientific and Medical Advisory Committee of the Coronary Prevention Group', *British Medical Journal*, 1987, 295, pp.1246-7.

23 The White Paper on Primary Care, *Promoting Better Health*, HMSO, 1987, adopted the fashionable idea of general practitioners as key workers in preventive care and health promotion, and amongst other changes, announced the abolition of free dental and optical checks. General practitioners may be becoming 'key workers' by default as other professional groups with similar claims, like health visitors, nurses or social workers decline or disappear under their workloads. Charging for preventive eye and tooth care whilst

adding to the workload of GPs seems an illogical approach to health promotion.

24 *Time to Care*, Secretariat for Futures Studies, Pergamon Press, 1984. These issues have been taken up by the Austrian Social Democratic Party and by the Italian left, but not by the British Labour Party. See also Laura Balbo and Helga Nowotny (editors), *Time to Care in Tomorrow's Welfare Systems: the Nordic Experience and the Italian Case*, Eurosocial, 1986.

25 The mass of evidence assembled and analysed in the Black Report showed that the health experience of the unskilled and semi-skilled working class relative to that of the managerial and professional class had worsened, even though overall population health had improved, in the post-war period. This finding applied to death rates of both men and women in the economically active age ranges, to perinatal mortality and for death rates in children between ten and fourteen. Pre-existing class differences in maternal mortality and in death rates in children aged between five and nine have not changed. Only in the death rates of children between one and four has there been a narrowing of the class gap. (Peter Townsend and Nick Davidson, *Inequalities in Health*, Penguin Books, 1982, pp.74-5) The persistence of these class differences was confirmed in the Health Education Council's 1987 report *The Health Divide – Inequalities in Health in the 1980s*, which also emphasised the damage done to physical and mental health by unemployment, and the particularly poor health of working class women.

26 See David Stone, 'Screen Fantasy', *New Society*, 11 December 1987.

27 George Teeling-Smith, 'Other Things not Being Equal', *Health Services Journal*, 4 Febuary 1988, p.149.

28 'Finite need and infinite resources' lacks credibility because, firstly, it ignores the 'demand' element in medical care, by which social and psychological factors influence use of services; secondly it assumes that 'need' is an objective quality and not the product of agreement between the needy and the (potential) provider, so denying the possibility that professional interest can shape 'need', and, thirdly, it exaggerates the availability of human resources whilst ignoring the necessity for training, supervision and direction of these new found resources.

29 Julian LeGrand argues that the NHS as an institution needs to be preserved precisely because it holds down government spending on health services better than any other available system, and criticises the government's encouragement for commercial medicine on the grounds that it 'would inevitably lead to an increase in doctors' incomes and other costs, which the NHS would be forced to match. A major expansion of private health care is a recipe for the kind of health care cost explosion that has bedevilled the rest of the developed world.' *New Statesman*, 29 January 1988.

30 As the NHS has moved centre stage, previously uninterested political actors have turned their attention to it. Not only has the ultra-left decided to wallpaper the nation's bus shelters with exhortations to 'defend the NHS', but weightier forces have spotted the bandwagon's possibilities. Leon Brittain, excluded from Cabinet influence after the Westland affair, joined the fray in early 1988 with a pamphlet, *A New Deal for Health Care*, in which he advocates a National Health Insurance Scheme to fund the NHS, with the opportunity for holders of private health insurance to opt out. (For an analysis of this, see Peter Davies, 'Another Voice Enters the Funding Debate', *Health Services Journal*, 18 Febuary 1988.)

31 The Conservatives have found dealing with the Pharmaceutical Industry through the Voluntary Pharmaceutical Price Regulation Scheme (VPPRS) very difficult. One the one hand the government is critical of the kind of public subsidy it must give to the drugs industry to maintain a high level of profit, while on the other the industry is a supporter of the Conservatives and a major

contributor to private sector growth. The tribulations of the VPPRS are discussed in Griffith, Iliffe and Rayner, op. cit., Chapter 7.

32 See Clive Froggatt, 'Biotechnology: Shaping the Future', in *The Medical Annual 1987*, editor D.J. Pereira Gray, IOP Publishing, 1987.

33 The cost of MRI is very high, partly because it is still at the experimental stage, with only 600 whole body MRI scanners operating worldwide, but its ultimate installation and running costs are unpredictable since the exact indications for its use instead of other, cheaper techniques have yet to be worked out. See R.E. Steiner, 'Nuclear Magnetic Resonance Imaging', *British Medical Journal*, 1987, 294, pp.1570-2.

34 One example of this is 'shockwave lithotripsy', in which sound waves are used to destroy stones in the kidney and gallbladder, and so avoid surgical operation. The technique has no associated mortality, unlike surgery, requires an average in-patient stay of only three days, and is 92 per cent succesful. It is being developed both in the NHS and in the commercial sector. (G. Das *et al.*, 'Extracorporeal Shockwave Lithoripsy: First 1000 Cases at the London Stone Clinic', *British Medical Journal*, 1987, 295, pp.891-3)

35 The commonest available 'biosensor' is used for measuring amounts of glucose in the blood, and is becoming an important tool to help diabetic individuals control their disorder. Future developments are likely to include biosensor tests for bacterial throat and bladder infections, and for alcohol quantities in blood or urine, but research and production have been hampered by lack of expertise and insufficient commitment to invest. (Charles Kingdon and Sean Newcombe, 'Engineers Have Designs on Biology', *New Scientist*, 30 April 1987)

36 Used in conjunction with biosensors to read data, such microchip technology allows simple biochemical analysis of blood at the bedside, at the workplace and in the local surgery or clinic. Other technologies are being miniaturised, with portable ultrasound machines already on the market.

37 Recording medical information about an individual is essential, yet is consistently badly done. Medical notes are all too often an 'anarchic, illegible, misfiled "pot pourri", in up to three volumes'. (See Julian Jessop, 'Storing up Problems on Access to Records', *Health Services Journal*, 26 November 1987, which makes a mockery of professional claims to continuity of care.)

38 One mathematical model constructed to measure the likely size of the future AIDS 'epidemic' gave highly variable results depending upon assumptions made about the incubation period of the virus and the percentage of infected people who go on to get full AIDS, even though the model itself was simplified by including the wholly artificial assumption that virus transmission stopped in 1986! (R.M.Anderson, *et al.*, *Lancet*, 1987, 1, pp.1073-5)

39 HIV screening, says the World Health Organisation in a discussion of screening applied only to international travellers, would be extraordinarily difficult to implement, would fail to prevent the spread of AIDS and would divert resources from educational programmes about AIDS and measures to protect blood and blood products (like Factor 8 for haemophiliacs) from contamination. At best, and at great cost, it might briefly delay the spread of the disease within or between countries. ('To Screen or not to Screen', *World Health*, December 1987, p.15)

Demands for population or migrant group screening for HIV represent a pre-rational search for someone to blame which has taken precedence over rational debate on how to protect ourselves, according to Kobena Mercer in 'AIDS, Racism and Homophobia', *New Society*, 5 Febuary 1988. There is increasing pressure within medicine, particularly from epidemiologists, for 'anonymous' testing on a mass scale. This would involve testing blood taken from people for other purposes – say, routine tests done in an outpatient clinic or GP surgery – but without identifying its source. The information derived would be of no benefit to individuals, who could not be identified at all, but would give an idea of the extent of spread of the infection. For a review of the arguments about screening and 'anonymous testing', see Steve Connor and Sharon Kingman, 'The Trouble with Testing', *New Scientist*, 28 January 1988.

40 See *HIV and AIDS in the United Kingdom*, Office of Health Economics, 1988; *The AIDS Virus: Forecasting the Impact*, Office of Health Economics, 1986; and R.M. Anderson and R.M. May, *New Scientist*, 26 March 1987.

4 Orthodoxies and Heresies

The standard socialist response to the crisis of health care is to urge expansion of the NHS to restore lost services and accommodate new developments. This will not work, because it addresses only part of the problem, and at best we can only use this approach as a short term solution to an immediate cash-flow crisis. The NHS crisis of 1987-88 was created by the Conservative government through the imposition on Health Authorities of cash limits set at levels below the level of the health service's internal inflation rate, and in that sense it was a political crisis not a financial one. The NHS was not in a crisis, but the Conservatives were – over the NHS. Extra funding is necessary to correct the over-application of cost-containment policies inflicted on health care by Thatcher's Cabinets, literally to buy time so that the major structural problems outlined in previous chapters can be addressed in a rational, non-dogmatic and democratic way.

As a justification for continued campaigning against the government, gathering the widest possible support to achieve a clearly defined objective and against a clearly defined (and easily isolated) enemy, this is an adequate approach. But we cannot leave it there, if only because the government will not permit the other issues to drop. What would we do if time were bought with extra funding? What practical ideas do we have to make health care part of economic renewal, as well as sensitive to the changing needs of our society, and flexible enough to incorporate technological changes that may transform medical practice faster than we think? And how can we achieve these objectives without creating an industry which develops its own momentum, and with it the potential to escape government financial control?

If we are honest we must admit that there are few plausible answers, of either a tactical or a strategic kind, emanating from the left, and certainly no package of ideas, practices and policies that could be the basis for a popular movement for renewal of the health service. On the contrary, much left-wing thinking is of an over-specialised nature, rooted in past approaches, and perceived as 'technical' and therefore a problem for experts by an essentially passive population. Where that traditional approach has been avoided, as it has by those strands of the women's movement that have extended into health politics via issues like fertility control and community action, new approaches and understanding have been marginalised by mainstream socialist practice, which has remained centred on the orthodoxies of a trade unionism that is locked into pay issues and political processes that can be deeply sectarian. The 'artificial' crisis within the NHS engineered by the Conservatives should be their downfall, but given the lack of a real alternative to Thatcherite ideas, values and economic policies it may be that the right will be able to restructure health care by default. If socialists wish to minimise Conservative impact and influence, rapid action and faster thinking are needed. First of all, we must accept that our model of health care is no longer sufficient, and must change.

Class Vendetta?

We might also need to think the unthinkable. If Thatcherism is not just a class vendetta against socialism, but also an attempt to reorganise and rebuild society in the interests of a capitalism that is undergoing substantial change, we may have to see Conservative initiatives as real attempts to deal with real issues in a real, if unacceptable, way. It is easier not to face this, but to negate Conservatism at every opportunity, to rebel against its ideas and conventions, and to equate socialism with a 'counter-culture' that rejects all that Conservatism is, including its whole political agenda.

When Tories say that the NHS is adequately funded, we insist that it is not, and in this situation we are right and have been so since at least 1983, if not 1948! But when they say that the health service cannot meet all the demands made on it, even those who have to try to satisfy demand, and go beyond demand towards meeting real need, are tempted to deny this truism because it comes from the unlovely mouths of greedy and amoral Conservative politicians. We are wrong, but dare not admit it. To do so might reveal the shallow foundations of the political culture which created and sustained the NHS in its first forty years as an undemocratic, clumsily bureaucratic welfare institution. And admission might also carry us towards the emptiness of the old Labour right, whose barons were never a match for the strategic thinking and political skills of the Establishment. Yet admit it we must, and when we do so our position may improve, since we can learn that the Conservative reaction to the twin crises within British medicine gives us clues about a more effective and more appropriate model of health care.

Thatcherism's Lessons

What can we learn about health care from Thatcherism? First, that Conservatism fears the key concept of the NHS, the gift relationship. Second, that it has no workable alternative concepts with any staying power. Third, that centralisation of power and decentralisation of responsibility for running health services – or promoting health – are complementary and not contradictory. Fourth, that individual enthusiasm and involvement, and personal investment, are keys to development and change. And, finally, that finding alternative resources for the promotion, maintenance and salvage of health is both necessary and possible.

The gift relationship has two important aspects that terrify Conservatism, particularly in its Thatcherite form. It demonstrates that a moneyless economy is both possible and more efficient than one based on cash-exchange, as well as being more just. And it is potentially infectious, threatening other areas of social and economic life.

The efficiency of the NHS, when compared with other countries' systems, appears in its low administrative costs, its overall low cost within the economy, its lack of waste, and its higher quality. The conclusions of Richard Titmuss's **study of blood transfusion services in countries with**

NHS-type or commercially based health services should be compulsory reading in the new school curriculum.

> On four testable non-ethical criteria the commercialised blood market is bad. In terms of economic efficiency it is highly wasteful of blood; shortages, chronic and acute, characterise the demand and supply position and make illusory the concept of equilibrium. It is administratively inefficient and results in more bureaucratisation and much greater administrative, accounting and computer over-heads. In terms of price per unit of blood to the patient (or consumer) it is a system which is five to fifteen times more costly than the voluntary system in Britain. And, finally, in terms of quality, commercial markets are much more likely to distribute contaminated blood; the risks for the patient of disease and death are substantially greater. Freedom from disability is inseparable from altruism.[1]

By an irony of history it is a government obsessed with market solutions to economic problems that has had to find extra public funds for people with haemophilia who have been infected by the AIDS virus, caught from a contaminated blood product, Factor 8, imported from the USA.

American imports can be less harmful. The opinions of US commentators who have made an in-depth comparison of American and British health services deserve an audience beyond academia:

> The dilemma that the United States and many other rich nations face is how to encourage patients and providers to weigh in a humane fashion the benefits and costs of medical care. Most such nations have laboriously created institutions that shield patients from out-of-pocket medical costs. Yet these very institutions, in association with technological change, are largely responsible for creating the problem of rising costs that many nations now seek to solve.[2]

The insurance systems that pay American doctors and hospital companies so very well whilst preventing most employed US citizens from becoming destitute through illness fuel the inflation in health care costs that worry government's lacking our advantage – a centrally controlled health service.

> Imagine ... an American President determined to hold national health expenditures to the current 11 per cent of GNP. What lever would such a President pull to accomplish this task? Tell the Congress to cut the benefits of Medicare and Medicaid? That would not force the congress to do anything, especially when the opposing party controls the legislature. But even if the policy were adopted, what is to prevent other medical spending from rising to make up for part of the shortfall? Or for private health insurance to fill in the gaps left by public choice? Or to stop the old and the poor either paying more or shifting their costs onto the bad debt ledger of health providers, to be made up from other payers?[3]

Britain's better structured health service also produces some results that are as good, if not better than, those of the USA.

> Overall, despite the economic straightjacket into which the NHS has been forced, Britain's health indices continued to improve in the 1970s and early 1980s and its remaining class differentials in health status are no worse, and in many ways better, than those in the US or in other countries where access to health care depends more heavily than in Britain on income, education, race and class. It is interesting to speculate on what the health consequences to Britain's population, with its high levels of unemployment and other elements of economic distress, would have been had they not had a functioning NHS to call on during this difficult period ... The NHS, for all its underfunding and other problems, remains in our view a model from which the US can learn a great deal.[4]

Proposals for health insurance, 'health maintainance organisations', internal markets, voucher schemes and even an earmarked health tax offer us systems that are more expensive and less efficient than the one that we have already.[5] Their only advantage lies in the contribution that they make to reducing the accounting problems of central government. Money not spent by the state is money not raised by borrowing or by increased taxation. Inefficiency and over-expenditure in the private economy are of no great interest to this government – at least, for the time being – and may even appear as growth in productivity of commercial industry, so bizarre is conventional economic thinking.

Worse than the economic superiority of the existing system is its subversive potential as a model for social activities and needs. If medical care can be freely available at the time of need, and paid for from the common wealth without the financial punishment inflicted on high users by insurance systems, why not apply the same principles to other necessities, like housing or transport? Both involve commodities where a finite need exists. Nobody can live in more than one home at any given moment, and very few people do nothing but travel. These needs can be measured, and arguably are much easier to measure than is the need for medical care. Even though demand for housing and transport varies, such demands can be satisfied by the one-off provision of a service (homes, transport systems) for long periods of time, unlike the need for medical care, which may vary substantially, unpredictably and very suddenly. In theory, an advanced planning mechanism operating in a stable economy could provide free housing and public transport for all citizens, if the political will permitted.

The Gift Relationship

The gift relationship is our great asset, delivering the goods in a material way through the everyday activity of the NHS, and promoting justice in the distribution of services (however imperfectly) through a mechanism that is more efficient than any of its potential rivals. Our task is to qualify the gift relationship in ways that allow us to overcome the legacy of past problems within the NHS whilst anticipating future developments in medicine, and in society.

The Conservative preoccupation with 'demand' points to the qualifications that we must consider, and brings us back to basic socialist ideas. If we all can make use of the common wealth, how can we know if we are using more, or less, than we should? The common wealth is finite, and others have needs too. How can any of us decide what is our, or anyone else's, 'fair share'?

We can argue that the dominant spirit in society must be one of restraint in using public health services, but this is a counsel of perfection with limited value, particularly in a society in which a generation or two has grown up with slogans like 'take the waiting out of wanting' as everyday commandments. Nor is it necessarily wise, since some people should be less restrained than they are in seeking help, in case the limited possibilities of medicine are lost because their particular problem has progressed beyond the point of repair. The class implications are also familiar. Too many have had no choice but to exercise restraint in so many aspects of life, whilst watching others indulge themselves in a growing range of luxuries, to make 'restraint' a popular new notion amongst working people. (If it has any ideological use, it will be to blame others for irresponsibility, in the way that some trade unionists disapprove of all strikes except their own.)

None of this may matter if the specific situation is clear-cut. The emotional responses of millions of people to appeals for funds for children's hospitals, the anger at the deaths of babies waiting (too long) for cardiac surgery, and the popularity of 'geewhizz' technology like CT scanners means that some problems will attract solutions whose costs few will begrudge. This is not necessarily a positive approach, for it must inevitably reflect a traditional view of what can, and should, be done, to the detriment of those who, for one reason or another, are seen as outsiders or undesirables. Health care for ethnic minorities, or for homosexuals, may earn the same low status as care of the mentally handicapped, or the elderly infirm, when the boundaries of the gift relationship are drawn by collusion between professional interests and conventional wisdom.[6]

Setting Boundaries

The gift relationship has boundaries, and we must accept that as a fact even if we argue amongst ourselves about where those boundaries lie. This has important implications. First, no matter how democratic the mechanism for setting priorities, someone somewhere will not accept the final judgement, and will want something else. People will seek alternative sources of health care, or do it themselves, or group together with others to create their own provision. This will give private medicine a residual and marginal function which we cannot avoid, and need not worry about. The idea of 'banning' private medicine is absurd because such plurality of belief, judgement and desire must always extend beyond the democratic consensus. In fact, we might gain more by thinking of ways of supporting a pluralistic approach to health care provision, provided that it promotes non-commercial solutions, than by brooding over the possible modifications of a decentralised apparatus.

'Alternative' medicine is in a similar position. Whilst much of it is right-wing chic, based on superficial thinking or theories that run well ahead of evidence, some of it is likely to lie on the collective side of the gift relationship boundary, and the political task is to distinguish between the valuable and the valueless, not to counterpose orthodoxy against 'alternatives'.[7] We need to think about charges to service users in the same way. Even if the technology exists to achieve a certain desirable but not necessarily essential objective, like the example of in vitro fertilisation discussed later, should it be freely used at the expense of other provision, or should the users make a direct financial contribution towards the costs of their care?

Setting Priorities

How, then, can we decide on priorities? The centralised structure of the NHS permits central priority-setting, and that is one of its advantages that we must preserve, but the experience to date suggest that it is not enough. The drift into commercial orthodox and 'alternative' medicine marks the escape of individuals from the priorities imposed by a state service. What part in decision-making and priority-setting in health services can socialists offer the whole population?

Once again we are short on answers. The idea of 'democratic control' reduces either to a wish for local government to regain control of health care or to schemes for electoral representation of health workers and the public on health service management bodies, whilst 'patient participation' remains a disappointing feature of primary care largely dependent upon the commitment and dominance of doctors, not service users. Each approach offers something, but neither gives a satisfactory solution. Local government control may appear as a dubious option, replacing the faceless bureaucrats of the DHSS with the local Town Hall bigots, and it revives the possibility of Conservative mismanagement of local services despite the intentions of national government. Whilst local politics has more significance for our everyday lives, even in an increasingly depoliticised culture, it still keeps the issues of control and choice of services at a distance from us as individual citizens.

Local 'patient participation' groups based on clinics or general practices may bridge that gap between policy and personal experience, even allowing for the powerful influence that professionals will have on these bodies, and for that reason their development should be a matter of concern for the left. Realistically, they are most likely to grow and prosper where the local traditions of community organisation coincide with a well developed ethic of community service amongst health workers. These features have no given political character, and may be working-class and socialist in some places but middle-class and conservative in others. Some 'patient participation' bodies may evolve into pressure groups for political change, but others may become adjuncts of the services, providing supplementary finance for the health centre or group practice through the usual methods of car boot sales and sponsored runs, and expressing an ethic derived more from charity than from collective responsibility.

Personal Responsibility

The missing element in socialist thinking is the idea and practice of personal responsibility. With so much socialist attention devoted to poverty, perhaps reflecting the guilt of the liberal intelligensia as much as the anger and despair of poor people, the idea of personal responsibility in health is undeveloped and so left open to absorption by the right. Of course, whilst for certain sections of the left the only reputable concern is for the inner-city poor, the idea of personal responsibility is meaningless. Only when we think of the employed and relatively well-off working class outside the inner cities, and the growing salariat of working-class origin, does the idea gain meaning. It is these groups that are attracted to the ideas of home ownership and share purchase, and who look towards the Conservative Party to introduce the social changes that will give them a greater stake in work and a greater degree of control over home life. The same offer applied to medical care makes personal health insurance an attractive idea. Whilst Conservatism does not follow Lenin's exhortation to let 'every cook rule the state', it does anticipate that all cooks can rule the kitchen, and a little beyond, even if they have yet to finish paying for it. Much of this shift of power is mythical, appearing in reality as a transfer of debt from the collective account to the personal mortgage, but it still allows individuals to escape from the 'democratic' alternative proffered by the left – political processes that can be confrontational, aggressive, unproductive and exhausting.

Collective and personal responsibilities are not contra-dictory, unless we are enthusiastic Thatcherites, and there is no rational reason for the left to ignore the personal dimension. Without a secure basis in collective provision, personal responsibilities cannot be exercised consistently. Ironically, the middle classes seeking their own interests through private health insurance are able to do so only because the NHS provides them with the safety net of a health service that is free and still far more comprehensive than anything that they can buy. They are unlikely to recognise that, but we can learn the lesson that they teach. A collective obligation to the individual is essential, but what should this mean for the future? And what are the individual's social responsibilities towards personal and collective health?

A Right to Health Care

The National Health Service does not promise to provide citizens with any specific service. Amazingly, ratepayers who froth at the mouth if the local council spends a few thousand pounds on some controversial project – not necessarily a centre for gays and lesbians, possibly just the planting of trees in a few streets – accept the expenditure of billions by central government on a health service whose functions are not defined in concrete terms. The regional variations in the availability of and accessibility to services are tolerated as if they were as uncontrollable as the weather.

This unthinking and uncritical delegation of power is out of place in a democratic society, and ending it may be one portal of entry to the difficult issue of democratic control of health services. We might benefit from thinking about the kinds of service that we actually needed, and codifying those needs into obligations upon Health Authorities. This will have two beneficial effects.

A range of legal obligations will simplify decision-making at local level, so that idiosyncratic influences are overcome and national standards of provision established. Even if the local Health Authority contains only born-again mone-tarists, it will have to obey the letter, if not the spirit, of the law. The function of the DHSS then becomes that of a standard-setter and inspector, rather than the hub of a centralised planning process. Local Health Authorities, however constituted, will be able to concentrate on the quality of the services that they provide, at which point the mechanisms for public involvement become important.

Secondly, the list of statutory services will be controversial, keeping health policy issues on the political agenda and directing debate about them away from issues of funding towards more complex arguments about value and priority. Because changing knowledge and technology will change possibilities for health care, the statutory obligations will need regular ammendment, forcing the left to treat health politics in a continuous way (as, for example, trade unions do with wage and salary negotiation) rather than in an episodic and campaigning manner. This will have important implications for politics itself. If the Conservatives are succesful in converting local government from a system of political control into an administrative apparatus overseeing privatised services, and in devolving planning powers to financially autonomous Health Authorities, arguments about health care financing will shift from centre stage, at the DHSS and the Treasury, to local stages, the (non-elected) Health Authorities themselves. We will then join other countries with mixed funding systems, in which conflicts on the scale of the disputes about the NHS in 1987-88 do not occur.

Aims and Objectives

We can now see that a range of new aims for the development of health care has become possible. A major objective of health policy, against the backdrop of statutory services, might be to increase individual ability to deal with health problems in the most appropriate context, whether that be home, school or workplace. Already the vast majority of episodes of ill health are managed by those experiencing them without recourse to professional help, except, perhaps, at the chemist. Those who seek help from the NHS get it from general practitioners, district nurses, health visitors and clinic staff, and only 5 per cent of those with an illness are referred for hospital care. The effectiveness of genuine health promotion policies can be measured. Instead of the government being proud of the 'productivity' of hospitals with a rising throughput, we might reasonably aim for:

> a reduction in consultation rates in general practice, with increasing consultation times;
> a shift from inappropriate use of medical resources towards a more appropriate use of a wider range of helpers, including nursing, midwifery, social work and psychology services;
> a shift of specialist services into the community, making access to specialist care easier and less costly to those needing it;
> a reduction in referals to hospitals for outpatient and inpatient care, and reductions in the numbers of some surgical procedures performed;
> the growth in numbers, size and influence of self-help organisations for people with particular health problems;
> decreased use of casualty departments for both emergency care and out-of-hours primary care;
> an increase in the number of agencies promoting and maintaining health.

These are not changes that depend upon an increase in preventive services or activity, but are the conseqences of rationalising the use of existing services by increasing the powers, options and choices of citizens. They would rely on different uses of information and information technology from those encouraged by a commercial culture, and emphasise the central importance to health of a wide range of social structures, not just the over-valued family.

Information Technology

Information technology offers us the chance to break through towards a participatory democracy, but a defensive and slightly paranoid left distrusts and fears it. The result is the predictable occupation of the whole territory of information technology by commercial forces. Videos on healthy eating can be bought at the check-outs of superstores, alongside the sweets and magazines on 'family living'. Diagnostic software that runs on home microcomputers can be bought in US newsagent chainstores, taking the user through the logical steps that reveal the likely causes of headache, backpain or sleeplessness, and their appearance in any country with a high per capita ratio of home computers is only a matter of time.

Unco-ordinated, hastily produced to occupy market niches, contradictory and confusing, these apparent improvements in health information may generate as many problems as they solve, but that is a poor reason for rejecting their approach. Why do we fail to see the possibilities of television and video, of computer-assisted diagnosis and learning, even of the telephone? The public libraries now becoming redundant could be renewed by this technology, allowing people to study information individually or in groups, in a flexible way, at their own pace, with or without 'expert' help alongside.

Information about the availability and character of health services is no less amenable to presentation on television newspages, but it has yet to appear amongst the weather forecasts and warnings about motorway traffic delays. What is to stop the NHS having a telephone advice service, like the immensely popular medical phone-in programmes of commercial radio, or the help lines set up by gay organisations to cope with AIDS and the fear of AIDS? Why not have one clearing number – 999 would do – for emergency medical services as well as other emergency assistance?

This should be familiar ground for the left, at least for Marxists educated in an understanding of the contradictions between the means of production and the relationships of production, but it is not. Catching up with new technology and its democratic implications is a major priority for socialists, who will need to run fast if they want to master the existing possibilities before the arrival and commercial exploitation of 'expert system' computer programmes and interactive television.

Personal Medical Records

We could go further, and try to use microchip technology to transform health care by one simple action – giving medical records to their real owners. Nothing new is needed to achieve this. Current computer software could allow an individual's whole medical history to be recorded on a pocket-sized plastic disc, which we could all possess and which we would be obliged to safeguard as a passport to medical services, just as we take responsibility for our passport for overseas travel. By using passwords and entry checks, the programme could be made to refuse all data entries that are not approved both by the record's owner and by someone with responsibility for health care, so that information stored would represent more of a consensus than do existing written records. Careful choice of computer operating system, language and disc would allow the record to be read on simple and widely available hardware.

The effects of introducing this one piece of information technology could be long lasting and profound. For the first time medical records would be coherent, comprehensible, structured, accurate and comparable, ending the era of the illegible, incomplete (or wholly missing), inaccurate, repetitive and disorganised written documents used in hospitals and clinics. For the first time the record's true owner would be able to read the record's contents and, if a user-friendly programme is used, understand them. Professionals wanting access to anyone's medical record would have to ask for it! No other comprehensive record need be kept in any part of the NHS on any individual, other than a back-up copy of the original.

Communication between different parts of the health

service could occur through the disc, abolishing the need for referral and reply letters, co-operation cards and duplication of test results. The record could become an educational resource for its owner and anyone else allowed access. Research would be possible using pooled records, but obtaining informed consent from the owner would become more than a formality, and the researchers need not be academics funded by government or industrial grants. Trade unionists looking for work-associated illnesses in a particular workplace could gain information from their members personally held medical records, assuming they could gain their confidence. A tenants' association suspicious about the unhealthiness of particular dwellings would have the same research potential, again subject to residents' approval and the availability of simple computing facilities. And every citizen would have an obligation to look after the most important piece of medical information there is – personal and family history – whilst being in a position to use that information in socially as well as individually responsible ways.

Autonomy

Information technology, deployed in the ways described, is a necessary precondition for the active involvement of citizens in health care, but is it sufficient for the growth of personal autonomy, that free development of each which must preceed the free development of all? Will new sources of information give even greater advantages to those already having the best deal? Can democratic practice be based on knowledge alone, and still meet everyone's needs? Or do we need to think of obligations that bind us as citizens, in the provision of health services as much as in the use of personal transport or the observance of civil law?

The gift relationship could assume a relationship of reciprocity between each citizen and the health service. At the moment it does not, but instead offers professional skills and judgements as the decisive factors that determine how health and illness are managed. The social obligation contained within the phrase 'to each according to need' is not yet balanced by the individual responsibilities inherent in the original opening words of Marx's definition of communism, 'From each according to ability, to each according to need'. Perhaps it should be. Why should we not think about individual obligations to maintain health? Why not consider making receipt of maternity benefit dependent upon attendance for antenatal care, as in France? Or making the immunisation of children against the main infectious diseases compulsory, as in the USA? Or only allowing free dental repair work if the individual can show that preventive dental care has been done regularly in the past, as was recently debated in Hungary?

This may seem an inappropriate or even dangerous attitude in a country in which an increasing number of people experience low income, poor housing and insufficient education, and also bear a disproportionate burden of illness, but that is a defensive response that carries a high political risk. First, the existing approaches to changing the status of the poorest sections of the working class, based on benign social engineering, have not succeeded. The poorest members of our society will have no more control over their own destiny because of the attentions of social workers or the construction of health centres. They may be slightly better off, but their status will not change. Some other answer must be sought, and the right offers its own 'trickle down' theory of wealth diffusing from the organised, competitive core to benefit the periphery of the disorganised and the 'less fortunate'.

We can reject the 'trickle down' view as absurd without returning to the somewhat weary model of state 'welfare'. At some point socialist thinking will need to focus on the strong currents of self-reliance present in different forms within the different strata of the working class, and seek ways of amplifying those currents. Those struggling to survive or bring up families on supplementary or unemployment benefit exist under harsher obligations than any discussed above, and know how to manoeuvre within a system that is hostile to them. Would they really be unable to cope with a floppy disc, or compulsory immunisations, in a society that concentrated its resources on homes, work and education? And will that better society come into existence without their efforts, including the take-up of habits and ideas that are prototypes of the new order?

Costs

If the future National Health Service is obliged to supply citizens with a guaranteed range of services, and citizens are obliged to use some of those services, costs are likely to rise because a backlog of work currently neglected will need attention. If every UK resident carries a personal medical record on a floppy disc, every NHS institution will need the machinery to read and write on the record. The capital and running costs of the NHS will rise and, as new uses are found for newly introduced facilities, spending will strain planned budgets. Will Britain's economy be able to afford it?

That depends in part upon political choices, and in part upon economic strategies pursued by whatever type of government succeeds the Conservatives. If the third of the scenarios outlined in Part 1 (Thatcherism defeated in 1992) is right, the economic situation may be better because money would be available to invest in the NHS, but the political will to invest it in appropriate ways may have been sidetracked into the campaign to defend the health service and remove the government. If either of the first two scenarios (prolonged Conservatism) are correct, economics may not favour the NHS because the damage done to manufacturing will be profound, but the political culture of the left will have changed and health care will be seen in different, and more realistic ways.

Whenever the end comes for Thatcherism a new government, socialist or otherwise, will need to reconstruct a ruined manufacturing economy, restore a dramatically delapidated social infrastructure and create a new international role for the nation. These are planned acts of enormous scope. The renewal of health services will be only one aspect of massive social change, and not the most important at that.

Industrial Growth

Re-industrialisation will be the most important health promoting action of the new government because it will reduce unemployment, increase GNP and per capita income, and supply basic materials for renewal of transport, housing and public health and medical care. How that industrial growth occurs will have an impact on future health and on health services themselves needs some thought. Rapid growth of manufacturing would require preferential investment in industry rather than services, need a substantial shift of resources into education and training to make up for the damage done by the Conservatives, and could possibly generate illness through unchecked use of potentially hazardous new technology and new products or overloading of unsafe transport systems. Investment in health services would probably attract much lower priority even though rising incomes would have to be paid partly in 'social wages' (like medical care) rather than money to prevent excessive importation of consumer goods.

An alternative approach, demanding a much smaller GNP growth rate, would involve freezing the real incomes of the employed, shortening the working week and limiting industrial development, so that jobs could be created without massive investment in manufacturing capacity, but with resource deployment into labour-intensive services like health care. Diminished needs for energy would improve the environment and promote health, by allowing the new government to close down nuclear power stations and reduce coal mining and consumption. New technology would not be introduced rapidly, but in a slow and controlled way with the aim of improving the quality of life rather than maximising GNP growth, so that the joining together of computers and telecommunications into a single yet differentiated national network would allow the technical development of health care discussed above at the same time as creating real jobs and permitting modest economic growth.[8]

Strategic Principles

Limited economic growth rates and planned redistribution would be the more favourable option for the renewal of the NHS, but in a consumer society with increasing inequality it may be the less likely outcome. Whatever the economic strategy adopted, policies for health care will be constrained by other, greater priorities for a considerable period. We need strategic principles that will guide NHS growth during that time, to offset the 'natural' tendency of medical services to determine their own priorities and direction. Some strategic ideas are available, both from UK and European experience. The Swedish Secretariat for Futures Studies suggests three preconditions for health care, which can be paraphrased as:

1. All policy is health care policy. Since living and working conditions, and lifestyle, do most to determine the need for medical services, they must have first attention, and policy developments in all areas must consider prevention of illness as a priority.
2. Whilst health care is fundamentally a communal responsibility, it is wasteful not to utilise and develop the competence of individuals for the provision of services. Many care tasks can be performed by non-professionals, including some tasks now done by paid employees and some not done at all. National and local government have the responsibility for ensuring that nobody is deprived of support and assistance.
3. To produce positive outcomes, civic influence over health service policy must increase along with individual influence over clinical services.[9]

A mechanism exists to put these principles into practice, in the 'life-cycle' welfare policies evolving in the Nordic countries. Scandinavian countries are approaching a situation in which the boundaries between work, family, education and 'welfare' (infirmity and retirement) are breaking down. Income is becoming separated from work throughout the life-cycle and not just at points in life where work capacity is limited, with the appearance of a *de facto* 'citizen's wage'. It is possible to have a high standard of living as a worker, a parent, a student or as a 'pensioner'. With reduced working hours for those in employment, and greater demands on citizens to contribute to caring services, this approach solves several problems. More labour is available for welfare services, at no extra cost beyond its training. Living standards rise, and with them health status. And those who make least use of, and get least benefit from, health services whilst paying most in taxation will be able to step out of employment to retrain or take on care responsibilities without losing out financially. This may contribute to the progressive political solution of the 'tax fatigue' that fuels the growth of conservatism throughout Europe.[10]

The next step in the development of 'life-cycle' welfare policies may involve the introduction of 'community service', an optional way of paying tax in labour rather than in money, so that a volunteer labour force can be recruited and trained for social care tasks in the same way that conscription is used to maintain armies. With this approach the gift relationship can be extended from the minimal gift of money collected as tax to the greater gift of work for others, chosen as a form of tax.

The Black Report

In the British context the Black Report (1980) contained a lengthy argument to justify changes in emphasis and policy towards welfare services and health care, although the left's preoccupation with the class inequalities catalogued by the report has overshadowed its programmatic conclusions.[11] Three objectives were identified:

> to give children a better start in life;
> for disabled people, to reduce the risks of early death, to improve the quality of life whether in the community or in institutions, and as far as possible to reduce the need for the latter;
> to encourage good health among a larger proportion of the population by preventive and educational action.

None of these proposals are new, but as a package they have important implications which the Black Report went on to explore. Firstly, top priority should go a comprehensive anti-poverty programme, with two components: a more just redistribution of resources; and the encouragement of self-dependence and a high level of individual skill and autonomy as the basis for creating a more integrated society.

Redistributive taxation is advocated, with the abolition of child poverty being its first objective. The Black Report argues that if the share of disposable income of the top 30 per cent were only moderately reduced, the sum available for distribution of social security benefits would be doubled. Even if we take a more pessimistic view of the amount of money that could be released by taxing the rich, and concentrate on relieving the 20,000 or so people who have £20,000 a year to spend on luxuries of their problem, the £400 million obtained each year is a significant sum if transferred to those in the greatest need.[12] The Black Report offers more, but at a greater political price, since it requires the reintroduction of progressive taxation to almost one third of the population, a group that has done very well out of Thatcherism. That will be a real test of socialist political skills and strategy.

For health care itself, the Black Report's plan includes a sub-strategy, a 'district action programme' that concentrates on the health of mothers and children, community care for the disabled and the elderly, health education focussed particularly on schools and on the organisation of a limited range of screening services. Ten areas with the highest mortality rates were picked out for exceptional, supplementary action by health and welfare services, both to reduce the burden of illness and to act as pilot studies to test new methods of working and measure the effectiveness of services. The Report's authors were conscious of the restricted amounts of money that could be made available, over and above the current level of spending on medical care, and opted for a carefully targeted scheme of new service development. Since we are likely to face the same, or greater, economic restraints we might now benefit from paying less attention to the bar charts of death rates and more to the political thinking within the Black Report.

A Sickness Service?

In particular, we could abandon the criticism of the NHS as a mere 'sickness service' that needs conversion into a real 'health' service. If the Black Report suggests nothing else, it locates the major cause of health inequality in material living conditions, with 'lifestyle' being of secondary importance and unequal distribution of medical services being a third factor.[13] The idea that there can be a health 'service' relects the dominance of professional thinking in popular culture, and leads directly into commodity relationships, since if 'health' can be made available by others' actions on us, it can also be bought.

Preventive medicine as a concept is a contradiction in terms, since medicine is necessarily responsive to disease processes, to deviations from the norm of healthiness. This response may be reactive, attempting to put right damage already done, and it may be proactive by trying to identify future problems and pre-empt further damage, but there is no sense in which it is primarily preventive in character. We need two, or perhaps three, different responses to ill health: first, active social policies that translate into real changes in working and living conditions, with all of us as participants with lesser or greater roles; second, assistance to all people who want to change some aspect of lifestyle like diet, smoking or alcohol consumption; and finally a high quality 'sickness service' that concentrates on the things now done badly – the early diagnosis of disease and the long-term support of people with long-term medical problems.

The NHS may have some contribution to the first response, by collecting accurate information about health and illness and by setting a good example towards its workforce and its users. Its workers may have a role in reinforcing existing trends towards healthier living, and may have some specific services to offer individuals unsure how to change their own behaviour, but there is no reason to believe that the NHS has a monopoly of wisdom or means. Even early diagnosis and long-term care, which should be the legitimate concern of the medical and nursing professions, are open to user involvement to a much greater degree than we believe.

A New Kind of Health Service

What kind of health service do we need and want, and what is possible? I want to suggest some possible features of a renewed National Health Service during a long period, I hope in the relatively near future, in which left-of-centre governments dominate politics.

1. Priorities for spending
Priority in health spending should be given to social services, not the NHS. It is realistic to aim to spend 8 per cent of GNP on health care – the EEC average – but for all

the reasons outlined before it would be both uneconomic and unjust to spend it all on extra medical services. Significant improvements in the quality of life of substantial groups of the population – the elderly infirm, the mentally handicapped, the disabled, and the mentally ill – depend on more extensive and better quality support services with maximum involvement of the service users and neighbourhood networks. The provision of childcare facilities will have more impact on the mental and physical health of parents – particularly women – than any quantity of tranquillisers or any number of psychologists, particularly if the users are involved in the provision of this care.

2. NHS spending
Within the NHS budget the first claim on extra resources after restoration of any essential services cut by the Conservatives should go to the lowest paid workers, to increase their spending power, their morale and commitment to the service, and to ease recruitment problems. Not all of these resources need to be payments in cash. Some could and should be improvements in living and working conditions, through the introduction of childcare services at the workplace, provision of better quality accommodation and subsidy of personal transport. There are two justifications for this concentration on the social wage aspect of increased personal income. A rise in disposable cash may set off a consumer boom that relies upon imported goods for its satisfaction, to the detriment of the economy. And the pay policy of the NHS should be one which emphasises the idea that important services should be available according to need.

Second claim should go to development of community-based services with the emphasis on preventive care; prevention of heart disease and strokes should be a high priority and become the subject of a planned approach that aims to modify clinical practice and make clinical workers accountable for their activities to the health service management structure. Renewal of buildings must be a lower priority, as it is now, with the only consolation being the availability of private hospitals suitable for acquisition. Some existing hospitals suffering from diseconomies of scale may need to be reduced in size to make them functional, the optimum size probably being about 500 beds.

3. Staffing

Overall staffing levels should be kept constant, particularly amongst doctors. There is little good evidence that we are under-doctored, and plenty to suggest that the NHS is unable to utilise its medical staff efficiently. The division of the service into parallel structures, the Health Authorities with their hospitals and clinics and the Family Practitioner Committees with their GPs, dentists, opticians and pharmacists, is fossilised history and needs breaking, even if this means loss of professional jobs or major shifts from work in hospitals to work in community settings. If nurse practitioners can do the same work as general practitioners at one quarter of the training cost and half the running costs, then a programme of professional replacement is necessary. If, as groups representing 'carers' have argued, there is only one nursing task that is not also done by lay people – operating-theatre nursing – then some of the work currently done by nurses could become the responsibility of community service workers paying their tax in labour. And if new technology permits 'bedside diagnosis' we should end the present reliance on large centralised hospital laboratories. Experimentation with these and other new approaches to delivering clinical care should be pursued with the aim of rationalising clinical practice in the most cost-effective way.

4. Cash limits

Budget restraints on Health Authorities should be maintained, and *appropriate* alternative sources of local finance encouraged as part of a strategy to renovate local economies through public enterprise. There is no reason why local industries should not buy packages of industrial health care from the NHS, under encouragement from trade unions. The NHS can sell its laundry services to other buyers – perhaps local authorities, perhaps privately owned nursing homes – and given some revolutionary changes in the kitchens, even become the centre of a commercial catering chain. Why should the NHS itself not develop new technologies as applied to medicine, given the investment capital? Such sources of new funds are appropriate because they permit greater local political involvement in service development and use a public industry – the NHS – as a springboard for local economic renewal. Flag-days and collecting tins do exactly the opposite, as does the desperate pursuit of money by District Health Authority managers suggesting that their Districts can service the commercial sector's own, natural market from within the overstretched resources of the NHS.

5. Pharmaceuticals

Concentration of all pharmaceutical production into one public industry will be necessary. This will permit the Department of Health to divert a proportion of the industry's profits into NHS services, to rationalise research and to use the industry's links with NHS professionals to promote government priorities in medical care. The existing private control of medicines production is a scandalous waste of resources, not only through non-essential competitive research spending, but also through valueless replication of drugs to obtain market shares and through massive advertising campaigns. It is time that we acted on Brian Abel-Smith's assessment of the pharmaceutical industry's approach to professional education:

> Expenditure on pharmaceutical advertising in both the UK and the US vastly exceeds the cost of continuing education for doctors in every aspect of practice. Indeed it is the failure to develop continuing education which makes genuine informative advertising necessary. For the costs of sales promotion activity in the United Kingdom, it would be possible for each general practitioner to have a teacher of medicine or therapeutics spend about a month a year working with him in his practice and giving him advice. A month would, however, be much more than would be required to inform a doctor about the five or six really valuable new preparations produced by the world pharmaceutical industry in a year.

Almost inevitably the health service would need fewer drugs than presently on offer, and the industry would contract during the public take-over, but that is a problem to be anticipated and planned for, not avoided. The political problems might be substantial, given the willingness of trade unions to collaborate with employers in defence of the industry, as the Association of Scientific, Technical and Managerial Staffs (now Management, Science and Finance – MSF) did over the government's introduction of a 'limited list' of prescribable drugs in 1983.

6. Charges

Principled objections to charges for services should be over-ruled. The costs of some services can be passed on to the user, at least in part, and our problem should only be in deciding on which few services attract a charge, and which are free. Present prescription charges are an unjust tax on the employed ill, generally fail to reduce medication use significantly and raise sums which could be obtained through rationalised prescribing. They should be abolished. Part of the cost of salvage work following injury in car accidents can be claimed from motoring insurance, and in a climate in which public transport is being promoted (on environmental, economic and health grounds), such claims could be increased. If an increasing number of young adults injure themselves through dangerous sports, should the NHS divert resources to assist them, or should they be asked to contribute to the costs of sports injury clinics through 'sports insurance'? And who should pay for in vitro fertilisation?

In vitro fertilisation is an important example, because it reveals the hidden assumptions about health care on the left. Those outraged at the thought of rationing access to IVF by price may ask what distinguishes a woman needing a lung transplant, a woman with broken legs, and a woman unable to conceive by any means other than IVF. The answers are simple. The woman needing a lung transplant is unlikely to get one since the technique is in its infancy and donor organs in short supply, and she is unlikely to survive it even if she is 'lucky' enough to be in the right place at the right time. If she has a preventable lung disease it might be right to ask why her deterioration was not prevented before rushing to heroic surgery. Through surgery the NHS will learn from her, and will get more from her than she gets from it. Knowledge of this may colour her judgements about accepting dramatic treatment.

The woman with broken legs is in a different category, since she will produce less and consume less of everything except services if her broken legs are not repaired. Following surgery that is relatively easy, well tried and effective she can continue to take part in every-day life as before, contribute to the production and reproduction of labour power at an optimal level and give the state legitimacy for its humane intervention. The infertile woman can claim no such need and no such combined economic and social significance (except when pronatalist policies are being pursued), since there is no obligation on her to have children. Unless feminists have been wrong all along, women do not have to meet a biological destiny through pregnancy; bearing children has become a choice not an obligation. The woman wanting a child by IVF therefore appeals for others to fund her desire, and it is reasonable to say that her desires should be left unsatisfied until others needs are fully met.

The desires of the infertile woman may be ranked equal to the needs of the injured woman or the woman with damaged lungs, but only if we adopt value judgements that deliberately permit this. There are many circumstances in which such value judgements can arise: the resources available to the health service may be abundant enough to allow both needs and wants to be satisfied; the birth rate may fall towards levels considered 'dangerous', so that child-bearing does become an obligation on the citizen; and an alliance of commercial and professional interests in IVF may be powerful enough to divert health service resources towards such programmes. At the moment the first and last circumstances apply. Professional power in the NHS is very much an issue of real estate – the control of beds and research facilities in hospitals – and IVF is as much an empire-building activity as a boon to the infertile. We may well have enough resources to support it, but rational debate about present and future priorities has not yet confirmed that.

Despite Bevan's dictum that 'the language of priorities is the language of socialism' we do not debate priorities openly, and the culture of the left almost prohibits any discussion of choices that are forced rather than free. This is not just an ideological failing, but also a consequence of practical problems which the example of IVF conceals. If we think about a woman who breaks her leg skiing in Switzerland and returns to the UK for treatment we can see the difficulties more clearly. She has injured herself through a voluntary activity that reflects her affluence. Should she be seen in the same light as the woman on supplementary benefit whose leg is broken in a fall down the unlit stairs of her tower block, the lift having failed yet again? There is a case for charging the skier some part of the cost of her treatment, which she can set against insurance. She has then truly taken the consequences of her desire to ski and not spread them across the whole community.

The victim of poor property maintainance cannot be held responsible for her injuries, but her landlord can, and there is a case for her to be treated freely and to be given help to claim damages from local government. This use of communal resources benefits her and the whole community, by restoring her to health and punishing negligence. However to accept this distinction sets precendents. Should climbers injured in the UK be treated on the same basis as skiers injured in Switzerland? And should others who injure themselves 'voluntarily' – for example, smokers with cigarette-related diseases – be penalised?

The left's usual response is to shout down any suggestion of overt discrimination and point to the injustice of insurance-based schemes that punish people for being ill through smoking, alcohol or other 'lifestyle' habits. Such insurance approaches are unjust, but that truth has been recruited to an illogical argument, since discrimination is occurring all the time within the NHS, and must continue to do so until a state of abundance is acheived. By having an open-door policy to medical care we are perpetuating demand-led services that are likely to favour the advantaged over the disadvantaged, the affluent over the poor, young over old and the 'normal' over the 'abnormal'.

There is no justice in the delayed treatment of elderly people needing hip replacement, the indifferent warehousing of the mentally ill and mentally handicapped or the perfunctory efforts at preventive medicine for working-class people. To correct those injustices we may have to discriminate against the skier flown back from Switzerland, if such sports injuries overburden existing and projected services, others with different sports injuries too. The decision has to be as much an economic as an ethical one, and it need not become a binding principle. Those whose illnesses are in some way related to past activities do not fit into the same categories, because habits like smoking and high alcohol consumption have social origins and physical aspects that override considerations of free choice. Many may claim to be addicted to skiing, but none are. Few may admit to being dependent on tobacco, alcohol or drugs, but many are. The point is that it is necessary to draw lines, and that we should do so consciously and openly.

7. Managing the health service
A new management 'culture' needs to develop, not on commercial lines as at present, but on a democratic basis emphasising widespread participation in day-to-day running of the service. Such democracy has advantages to health service managers. The wider the involvement, the wider the understanding that not all needs can be met immediately, and that not all wants are justified. Old concepts need decanting into new structures that make a reality of public ownership by extending the responsibilities of ownership to an ever widening population. The existing administrative structure of the health service is adaptable, and another costly and disruptive management reorganisation seems unnecessary. But existing workstyles will have to change, to incorporate the expertise of service users into planning and administration.

Every District Maternity Services Committee will need an input from local women's organisations, and those organisations will need resources to allow them to canvass user opinion in a comprehensive way. Every Primary Care Planning Team will need regular communication with clinic- and surgery-user groups, which will in turn need the personnel and funding to grow independently of benign professional paternalism. These and other changes in administration will need a cadre of committed, enthusiastic and democratically inclined managers. The Griffiths reform may have failed to produce anything like that, but we

should not confuse the principle of general and unit management introduced by Griffiths with the tasks imposed upon it
by the government, or the people drafted into post by the
DHSS.

Whilst a new, reforming government will need to replace
all the political placemen and women occupying key posts
in NHS administration, and all the dozy voting fodder
enrolled onto Health Authorities to support Conservative
policies unthinkingly, the powerful positions of manager
should be retained. They can still become agents for
reaching a wider consensus, and in a political culture
unaccustomed to participation the probable initial shortage
of activists for working democracy will enhance the role of
individual managers.

8. Statutory obligations

The first obligation on citizens might be the responsibility
for safeguarding the medical records of their children,
carried on floppy disc or 'smart card' (see Appendix A).
Other obligations need to be discussed, with the left taking
the initiative in the debate and using the existing channels
of communication through unions and community organisations to research public thinking and attitudes. 'Labour
Listens' may be a poor campaign but it could make a
powerful form of routine political work.

Central government must ensure that services meet
people's needs, by legislation to introduce 'Patient's Rights'
(statutory obligations on Health Authorities) and by
strengthening the Department of Health so that it can
enforce strategic direction upon elected Health Authorities.
Ideas for such a charter are outlines in Appendix B. The
new management culture will be needed to extend this
directive approach down to the working units of the NHS,
to ensure that extra resources are used effectively.

One dimension of such direction will be the continuation
of careful budget controls at every level of the health
service, but another one that is neglected by the
Conservatives will be the adoption of targets for health
care, like those proposed by the European Region of the
World Health Organisation and based upon the WHO's
charter, 'Health for All by the Year 2000' (see Appendix C).

9. Inequalities in health

Evidence accumulated since the publication of the Black Report in 1980 tends to support its view that some class differences in health are widening.[14] The primary objective of the NHS should be the progressive reduction in class inequalities in health (and in access to appropriate medical care). The targets will be preventable disabilities and premature death, with the emphasis on the extra burden carried by the working class. These objectives will not be achieved if people do not understand them, and the methods needed to reach them, and that will require a process of involvement and education beyond any currently practiced.

This shift towards preventing illness is unlikely to occur through the NHS alone, at least on any significant scale, for all the reasons discussed above, even though the NHS will have a small but important part to play. The primary actors in changing the material circumstances and everyday existence of people most at risk must be the bodies that express working-class aspirations and needs, whether they be trade unions, tenants' and residents' organisations, pensioners' groups or the British Legion.

If stress is a significant contributor to heart disease then it is as much up to unions to campaign against stressful working conditions as it is up to government to support them through legislation and through the efforts of the Health and Safety Executive. If workers in a particular industry want an on-site service to help individuals stop smoking, or control alcohol consumption, that is a legitimate objective for trade union activity and a facility to be introduced as part of that industry's social wage. Changes of this kind are likely to be much more significant in mobilising support for 'healthy living' policies and in producing real, lasting changes in health than any shift towards prevention and community services within the NHS, however necessary that is. We will have to tolerate divergence, not convergence of all functions upon one structure, within health care provision if we want to see rapid change and recruit large numbers of people into the 'caring' workforce.[15]

Taking the Consequences

What would all this mean for a new government, inheriting not only the economic problems created by Thatcherism but also the attitudes, values and institutions that it has generated? The consequences of the kinds of policies outlined are unlikely to cheer those whose socialism depends on the all-giving state or even the notion of a 'caring society', but perhaps we should interpret much current socialist thinking as a sub-genre within nostalgia, and look to future needs.

Amongst the practical actions and political problems of the new government we should anticipate:

> Further reductions in the numbers of hospitals and hospital beds of all kinds, with an increasing workload being undertaken in day-care units and in people's homes. New technology will come to the aid of the health service here, as will the outward shift of specialist care to the community.

> An incomes policy within the NHS that restrains higher professional salaries and narrows income differentials. Since commercial medicine in some form is likely to persist, income restraint within the NHS may encourage even more 'moonlighting' into the private sector. There are ways to minimise this, perhaps by making working conditions within the NHS substantially better than anything the diminished network of surviving commercial hospitals could offer, or by imposing penalties on some categories of staff if they use part-time status to work in rival institutions.

> Rivalry between the public service and commercial medicine might be advantageous to the renewed NHS, since it would offer some scope for the development of 'life-cycle' welfare within the health service itself. Part-time working could become the norm, for example, and repeated opportunities to retrain within and between disciplines could be made possible as a matter of course. There may be much to be gained by encouraging experienced health workers of different backgrounds to retrain in medicine, since they may well make much better and much more democratic

doctors than the current cohorts of high-achieving eighteen year-olds from 'good' schools.

Persistent rationing of services, with a strengthened barrier (in the form of extended community-based services) between the population and some forms of specialist care, and continued waiting-time between identification of a problem and its resolution. Whilst rationing will be unavoidable for some services, at least in some places, overall improvements in management and planning should reduce the differences in waiting times that currently exist between Health Authorities, and over time health promotion pursued with enthusiasm at community and workplace level should reduce the incidence of illnesses attributable to smoking and over-consumption of alcohol.

Transformation of professional roles, with people having more limited access to doctors but much more access to non-medical staff – nurses, counsellors, social workers and psychologists – working in the front-line. This is bound to produce friction, both amongst professionals and between them and service users, but the overall extension of choice and the increased opportunity for personalisation of services should be enough to offset the problems.

Continued growth of small-scale private medicine in many forms, with limited scope for restraint by government action. Realistically, a left-wing government could hope only to isolate and undermine commercial medicine, particularly where US multinational and local finance capital are involved, but not diminish 'cottage industry' private practice amongst either orthodox or alternative practitioners.

Delays in the introduction of new techniques whilst they are tested for value by a new Committee for Technology Assessment, and whilst other priorities are being dealt with. Constant assault on the quality of the NHS by those wanting faster innovation – commercial interests, some professionals, users expecting 'magic bullets' – will ensure that medical care remains a highly politicised issue, even though the devolved administration introduced by the Conservatives is maintained and transferred to local government control.

Conclusions

This scenario offers us a public health service that will become less demand-led and more provider-led as its relatively limited spending programmes unfold. Private provision will continue and individual use of it may even increase as commercial investment in its most organised forms diminishes, if only because old attitudes within the population clash with new forms of health service organisation, to the benefit of professionals underpaid or even unemployed because of the policies of the new government. The most important growth area will be in the resources and powers of local government, and there will be increasing scope for politics to influence the character of the local services that affect the health of local people. New opportunities will appear for the left to influence the growth of health care as health service management is opened up to democratic control, and local economies could be transformed as the NHS – already the major employer in many areas – comes to dominate provision of technical services to small-scale, privately owned businesses.

The structural changes within health care will reflect the continuing conflict between commercial and socialised medicine, but the working principles of the new public service will prefigure a new society. Through the health service individuals will be able to control information and to contribute to the provision of services and the deciding of priorities, in a way that is denied by the market. Workers within the health service will be able to change their jobs, to alter their working hours and to earn a worthwhile social wage as well as a cash income. Marx's vision of the breakdown of the division of labour had in it a person who hunts in the morning, fishes in the afternoon, rears cattle in the evening and is a literary critic after dinner, without ever becoming a hunter, a fisherman, a herdsman or a critic. We have a better prospect than this collection of solitary occupations and hobbies. By rebuilding the NHS on the foundations of user involvement and new technology, we can talk of an individual earning a citizen's wage for childcare in the morning, having a paid part-time job as a clinic nurse in the afternoon, teaching use of computer diagnosis 'expert systems' over the local interactive television network in the early evening, without pay, and still having enough energy and enthusiasm to enjoy others' company after dinner. Just as the foundation of the National Health service suggested that a socialist society could be created in post-war Britain, so a future health service could help extend the gift relationship into wider society.

This is a very long way from Bevan's dream and some distance from the compromise he cobbled together in 1948, but it will be a turning point in the development of public medical care and an escape from the unjust and ineffective mess of medical services that Thatcher's governments will bequeath on the nation. Not all medical services will be entirely free to the user, but the vast majority that are will be dealing with the serious problems of a society in transition from the backwardness of a market economy to the prosperity and stability of a planned one, and they will work well. Critics will be able to point out that the new National Health Service does not provide everything that is available in other countries under the heading 'health care', but socialists will be able to reply that it neither could nor should do so. And money will come from different directions in different places, ending the pretence of a tidy monolithic institution.

If this happens we will be in debt to the Conservatives for the instability they once inflicted on the biggest institution in Europe outside the Red Army, and also on the traditions of the British left.

Notes and References

1 Richard Titmuss, *The Gift Relationship: From Human Blood to Social Policy*, Allen & Unwin, 1970, p.246.
2 Henry Aaron and William Schwartz, *The Painful Prescription: Rationing Hospital Care*, The Brookings Institution, 1983, p.134.
3 Ted Marmor, 'Health and Efficiency', *New Society*, 5 Febuary 1988.
4 Victor and Ruth Sidel, *A Healthy State: An International Perspective on the Crisis in United States Medical Care*, Pantheon, 1983, pp.174-5.
5 The 'internal market' idea, for example, has been pursued since the publication of a report on the NHS by American health economist and Pentagon adviser, Alain Enthoven, by the Nuffield Provincial Hospitals Trust in 1985. Enthoven argued that the District Health Authorities should become autonomous trading bodies, selling their services to each other at market prices. Despite support for

this from some London teaching hospitals, the Alliance (as was) and the *Economist*, the idea was poorly received, at least until the Carlton Club seminar in 1987, because of its obvious faults. Money would be circulated, but no new resources would appear; and compensation for cross-boundary flows of workload is built into current budgeting and occurs anyway, but is retrospective. (Jolyon Jenkins, 'Take Up Your Bed and Walk to Market', *New Statesman*, 20 November 1987)

6 The government's next steps in combatting the spread of AIDS remain to be seen, but Clause 29 of the Local Government Bill, which seeks to prevent local councils from promoting gay activities, may turn out to be a greater obstacle to the develoment of an anti-AIDS strategy than the moral condemnation of the far right. Homophobia can now be expressed through greater efforts to weed out the potentially infected, including requests from insurance companies to general practitioners to report on the likelihood of risk of infection, and on any history of sexually transmitted disease, of insurance applicants. AIDS testing is being introduced into routine medicals for new employees of Texaco, on the grounds that the company automatically enrolls employees in the company pension scheme and accepts only those of average risk. If these practices spread then those carrying the virus may be unable to get a job to pay the mortgage for which they will not be eligible! The motivation for seeking testing on health grounds is likely to be reduced by such social ostracism, with the result that some individuals who will benefit from help will delay their search for it. Since having an AIDS test, regardless of result, seems to be more effective in persuading high-risk people to change their sexual habits than is counselling, an opportunity for important preventive care will be lost. (Jeremy Laurence, 'AIDS: The Politics of Panic', *New Society*, 22 January 1988)

The transfer of resources to institutional care of the mentally handicapped has been both modest and slow, despite a succession of scandals over patient care, and is in marked contrast to the rapid change that has occured in the delivery of maternity services, with the virtual eradication of community-based services by hospital-centred ones despite the absence of good evidence to justify such a shift. (For a detailed review of official enquiries into service failures in long-stay mental illness and mental handicap units, and the significance of the low priority accorded to this field and the isolation of its workers, see J.P. Martin, *Hospitals in Trouble*, Basil Blackwell, 1984.) More recent shifts from institutional to 'community' care seems to have involved economic rationalisation of resources rather than the development of alternative forms of care, and the intended transfer of responsibility for service delivery from the NHS to local authorities has been limited and inadequate. (Joanna Ryan and Frank Thomas, *The Politics of Mental Handicap*, Free Association Books, 1987, Chapter 8) Whilst in the short term 'community care' is cheaper than in-patient care, in the longer term adequate quality community care is more expensive, but also more desirable. (Stuart Etherington and Nick Bosanquet, *The Real Crisis in Community Care*, GMPH publications, 1986)

7 See David Armstrong, 'The Problem of the Whole Person in Holistic Medicine', *Holistic Medicine*, 1986, 1, pp.27-36.

8 The advantages and disadvantages of these 'growth' and 'green' options for future development are discussed in detail in Bob Rowthorn and John Wells, 'Towards 2025', *Marxism Today*, November 1987, pp.36-9. The 'third technological revolution' based on robotics, services organised through interactive terminals and on-demand information retrieval and its impact are discussed in Daniel Bell, *The World in 2013*, *New Society*, 18 December 1987.

9 *Time to Care*, Swedish Secretariat for Futures Studies, Pergamon Press, 1984, Chapter 7.

10 See Gosta Esping-Anderson, 'Life Cycle Policy as the Emergent Model of

Scandinavian Welfare States', in *Time to Care in Tomorrow's Welfare Systems: The Nordic Experience and the Italian Case*, Laura Balbo and Helga Nowotny (editors), Eurosocial, 1986.
11 Peter Townsend and Nick Davidson, *Inequalities in Health* (The Black Report), Penguin Books, 1982.
12 Alec Nove, *The Economics of Feasible Socialism*, George Allen & Unwin, 1983, pp.156-7.
13 This is not new either, but the argument has always been resisted by clinicians, who with some justification saw it as a rationale for refusing to fund services deemed essential by those actually responding to demand. That resistance has not helped, since other rationales can be found by those needing them, and NHS workers defending their service are drawn into the trap of appearing as little more than advocates of their own clinical speciality and their own narrow interests. (See Thomas McKeown, *The Role of Medicine*, Basil Blackwell, 1979, for an extended analysis of the relative importance of material environment, social activity and medical services in shaping health and illness.)
14 This evidence is reviewed in Richard Wilkinson (editor), *Class and Health: Research and Longitudinal Data*, Tavistock, 1986.
15 This process is under way. Although half of Britain's workforce and 80 per cent of workplaces have no access to even basic occupational health services beyond first aid, a survey of workplace health activity, policies and underlying influences between 1976 and 1986 found that:

> The focus of workplace activity had shifted during the decade. Occupational disease production is seen as important as accident prevention. Priorities for future development include action against noise, dusts and accidents, then exposure to chemical hazards or to agents causing cancer or genetic abnormalities.
>
> Increasing attention is being given to general health promotion, with issues like smoking, alcohol and stress getting as much emphasis as major occupational hazards. Diet and cancer screening are seen as priorities for future activity, and there is growing recognition that the workplace has a wider role in promoting health amongst workers whether the factors affecting it originate inside or outside the workplace.
>
> The major influences on workplace health activity have been government legislation and pressure from within the workforce. Independent health promotion bodies have been of much less significance.
>
> The major resources to assist future activity are seen to be government funding and information on succesful programmes.

(Tony Webb, Richard Schilling, Penny Babb and Bobby Jacobsen, *Health at Work*, a report on Health Promotion in the Workplace for the Health Education Council, 1986)

With the present government extra funding seems unlikely, and trade unions will need to look elsewhere for resources. Information exchange is a less daunting issue, and a point at which NHS workers can make an immediate contribution, both at local level through trades union networks and through national level, through the TUC and specialist 'work hazard' organisations.

Appendix A

Outline of Personally Held Medical Record

This is the outline of a personal medical record held upon a protected floppy disc. The programme assumptions are:

1. Wordprocessor, graphics, database and spreadsheet facilities operate as a single programme;
2. Standard datafiles, graphics and spreadsheets of, for example, normal growth rates in children or ranges of weight-for-height in adults are 'read only';
3. Data entry requires two 'passwords'; the record owner and that of the health worker entering data (this could be the registration number with the General Medical Council, for a doctor). Passwords could be entered manually at a keyboard or using a personal identification number encoded on a plastic card, to be read by machine only;
4. Data will be encrypted at entry, and compressed to save disc space;
5. Sensitive data can be hidden further in protected files with limited access for both reading and writing;
6. Automatic date and time logging cannot be changed without the two passwords used to enter that piece of data;
7. Subprogrammes within the core programme will be activated by unauthorised interference with the record and damage existing data.

The record could contain the following files:

Family History

(The parents' health summaries copied from their records, plus a family tree from each parent, also copied from their discs.)

Maternal Maternity History

(Also copied from the mother's record.)

Birth Data

(All information about the individual's birth.)

Growth and Development

(Background graphs of 'normal' growth, upon which individual growth can be plotted; and a developmental checklist upon which actual development can be written.)

Prevention Card

(A checklist of all standard preventive measures to be taken over a lifetime, and a record of those actually done; this record would need to be adaptable, as new preventive approaches become available. This record should contain risk factor measurements like blood pressure and weight-for-height (expressed graphically as the Body Mass Index) as well as details of immunisations. Other 'normal' data would be useful, like a graph of lung function upon which individual measures can be plotted.)

Running Record

(A free text record of all contacts between the record's owner and the health service, containing details of medical, dental, nursing and other professional contacts organised into files that can be read in groups (all dental consultations, for example) or in chronological order, with subcategories for reports and investigation results, and a capacity to identify key information that can be exported to a Summary Sheet. Automatic transfer of factual data –

blood pressure, weight, lung function – to the Prevention Card would be useful, as would the capacity to show separate measurements of, say, iron levels in the blood graphically.)

Planning Template

(A plan for future health care which acts as a reminder to the owner and to health wokers of important tasks, targets or objectives.)

Occupational History

(Giving details of all occupations, with the emphasis on identifying known work hazards.)

Social Situation

(Containing details of accommodation, marital status and own family relationships, with a family tree that can be copied to an offspring's record or to update that in Family History.)

Maternity History

(Including details of each birth, and of the baby's health in its first week of life, plus any significant medical events in the child's life that may be relevant to future maternity care.)

Summary Sheet

(A chronological summary of major medical events and significant background history, with key information copied from other files automatically.)

No record can be made entirely secure, and since personal access to personal information is one of the primary objectives of this system, obstacles to reading data would be undesirable. To prevent falsification of data the record can be protected by demanding passwords for entry, by use of a double password 'key', by encrypting information, and by using hidden files for specific information. Two copies of each record would be needed, one held by the owner and the other kept as a reserve with the main service provider – in the present context, the general practitioner – who could cross-check information. The use of a subprogramme to detect and pre-empt unauthorised interference with data (in effect, a benign 'virus') would act as a deterrent to record falsification.

Appendix B

A Patient's Charter

The 1986 Annual General Meeting of the Association of Community Health Councils of England and Wales adopted the following Patient's Charter as a statement of principles and a framework for further consideration of the rights and responsibilities of patients and health care providers.

All persons have the right to:
1. health services, appropriate to their needs, regardless of financial means or where they live and without undue delay;

The report of the AGM published by ACHCEW noted that this is already an established 'right'. It is, however, vague and allows ample scope for interpretation of 'appropriate', 'needs' and 'undue'. Perhaps a Patient's Charter should specify statutory services for all Health Districts, including: a right to maternity care with a choice of places of birth; an integrated child health and development service with a presence in schools as well as in the locality; contraceptive and family planning advice, including a day-care unit for early termination of pregnancy in every District; easy access to an early diagnosis service based in the community with named specialist services with in-patient facilities at District and Regional level; 24-hour nursing care in the community, including community hospitals and home care, drawing upon the experience of 'hospital at home' pilot schemes. (see Freda Clarke, *Hospital at Home*, Macmillan, 1984); and a personal medical record with back-up copy held at the locality clinic.

2. to be treated with reasonable skill, care and consideration;

This has implications for: staffing levels, particularly in hospital nursing where work is most intense; educational programmes, especially in medicine where the mismatch between what is taught and what is done is so great; and in the provision of services for ethnic minority groups.

3. written information about health services including hospitals, community and general practitioner services;

To which we can add that in a 'wired society' information should be available on all commonly used media, including teletext.

4. register with a general practitioner with ease and to be able to change without adverse consequences;

5. be informed about all aspects of their condition and proposed care (including the alternatives available) unless they express a wish to the contrary;

The slippery concept of informed consent is reviewed in Carolyn Faulder, *Whose Body is it?*, Virago, 1985. This book includes details of the American Hospital Association's Patient's Bill of Rights and the European Parliament's 1984 resolution for a European Charter for the Rights of Patients.

6. accept or refuse treatment (including diagnostic procedures) without this affecting the standard of alternative care given;

7. a second opinion;

8. the support of a friend or relative at any time;

9. advocacy and interpreting services;

10. choose whether to participate or not in research trials and be free to withdraw at any time without affecting the standard of alternative care given;

11. only be discharged from hospital after adequate arrangements have been made for their continuing care;

12. privacy for all consultations (and examinations, particularly with the growth of video-recording as a teaching technique and also as a way of recording data);

The video disc makes it possible, in theory, to record consultations, examinations, investigations and operations as part of the individual's medical record;

13. be treated at all times with respect for their dignity, personal needs and religious and philosophic beliefs;

14. confidentiality of medical records relating to their care;

The ACHCEW report noted that this was an established 'right' which was not actually observed since medical records are readily accessible to NHS staff other than those working directly with the individual. Computerised medical records can be designed to protect information and only allow access to those with passwords or identification numbers. Although such records are not perfectly safe, entry to them is harder than entry to the average general practitioner's surgery.

15. have access to their own health care records;

16. make a complaint and have it investigated thoroughly, speedily and impartially and be informed of the result;

17. obtain an independent investigation into all serious medical or other mishaps whilst in NHS care, whether or not a complaint is made, and, where appropriate, adequate redress.

Implications for Britain of Targets for the European Region of the WHO

The targets below have been identified by the Faculty of Community Medicine of the Royal College of Physicians in order to achieve the European 'Health for All' goals by the year 2000.

Each Health Authority will need to devise and pursue its own targets and strategies, working in partnership with other organisations and members of the local community.

A feasible set of targets might be:

by 2000, ensure greater equality in health:

> where differences exist between geographical and or socio-economic or ethnic groups in the incidence and mortality from specific conditions these should be reduced by 50 per cent by securing an improvement for the disadvantaged group.

By 2000, achieve health related goals which:

> add life to years, by ensuring the full development and use of physical and mental abilities;
> add health to life, by reducing disease and disability; and add years to life, by reducing premature death.

These can be achieved by:

> reducing the prevalence of mental illness to the extent that there is a 25 per cent reduction in the prescription of hypnotics, sedatives and tranquillisers;
> reducing by 10 per cent the prevalence of severe mental handicap;

reducing by 15 per cent the prevalence of severe physical handicap at birth and as a result of accidental trauma;

reducing by 50 per cent the incidence of stroke by the prevention and control of hypertension;

reducing by 50 per cent the prevalence of total tooth loss in adults (this may be one of the most accessible targets since there is already a reducing prevalence of caries);

reversing and then reducing the rising incidence of sexually transmitted diseases;

reducing by at least 25 per cent the number of unwanted pregnancies, particularly amongst women aged less than twenty years;

reducing by at least 15 per cent the mortality, and disability, from such specific preventable infections as measles, pertussis and congenital rubella (it may be possible to eradicate these diseases entirely);

maintaining a low level of maternal mortality;

reducing by at least 20 per cent the perinatal mortality rate;

reducing by at least 20 per cent the infant mortality rate (both these rates are much higher than in many other European countries; a sustained and co-ordinated campaign is required to reduce hazards to the child in utero and the premature onset of labour, as well as to ensure that maternity services respond sensitively to the needs of their patients);

reducing by at least 20 per cent the mortality rate from all causes of accident at all ages;

reducing by at least 20 per cent the mortality rate from cancer in those aged less than 75 years;

reducing by at least 30 per cent the morality rates from both stroke and heart disease in those aged less than 75 years.

By 1990, develop a health service structure which:

ensures that all its staff understand the contribution they can make to the achievement of local targets;

encourages the health service to make a contribution to policies in other sectors which promote healthy lifestyles and reduce health hazards;

enhances the role of the family and other social groups;

provides appropriate levels of service, including efficient initiatives for the prevention and early detection of ill health, which are distributed according to need and are both acceptable and accessible; incorporates an active programme of health education.

By 1990, ensure that the environment provides

protection from:
toxic compounds;
hazardous wastes;
ionizing radiation;
contaminated foods;
harmful food additives;
hazards at work;
harmful biological agents;
other harmful substances and influences;
suitable housing for all;
safe water supplies;
safe disposal of human, household and industrial waste.

By 1995, achieve for the local community

a healthy diet;
physical fitness from appropriate regular exercise;
effective and acceptable control of fertility;
sound dental hygiene in children and adults;
improved immunisation uptake levels for:
pertussis to 80 per cent by age one year;
polio, tetanus, diphtheria to 90 per cent by age one year;
measles to 90 per cent by age two years;
rubella to 95 per cent of girls by age fourteen years;
a reduction in mean blood pressure levels;
a reduced prevalence of obesity;
a reduction in smoking to 25 per cent of the adult population and a negligible rate amongst school leavers;
a reduction in alcohol and drug misuse and self-poisoning.

Index

also available

Banking on Sickness

Commercial Medicine in Britain and the USA

Ben Griffith, Steve Iliffe and Geof Rayner

Privatisation poses a major threat to the National Health Service. What is not so well known is the variety of ways in which individuals and companies operate for profit within the NHS. From doctors and consultants taking on private medical work to the contracting out of hospital cleaning and other services, from the massive profits made by the drug companies to the ambiguous position occupied by opticians, dentists and others, there are numerous ways in which commerce invades health care.

The Thatcher years have witnessed a major growth of private health insurance and US-owned private hospitals and clinics which subvert the egalitarian principle on which the NHS was founded. Meanwhile, 'private' but non-profit medicine in the area of pregnancy and abortion services continues to play an invaluable role.

The complexities of commercial medicine are explored in this clear and lucid book, the first to examine a crucial aspect of commercial medicine. *Banking on Sickness* is essential reading for health service workers and all those worried about the future of health care in Britain.

'Considerable food for thought ... an interesting and thoughtful discussion about the compatibility of private (or commercial) medicine with a tax free-funded health service ... Obviously this is a book which many colleagues will buy only to burn or to hurl through windows' – *Lancet*

'This informative and timely book ... pulls together a wealth of valuable facts and arguments.' – *City Limits*

£6.95 paperback